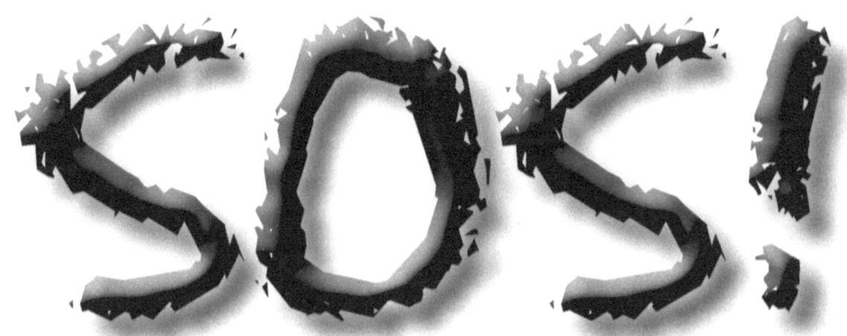

my child is always sick

Discover if your child has food allergies

Maria Alejandra Gonzalez

First edition: December 2009

Second Edition: June 2012

ISBN-13:978-1479124909

ISBN-10:1479124907

Second Edition

To my husband and my children

TABLE OF CONTENTS

INTRODUCTION

I decided to write this book because I could not keep quiet about all that I have discovered in recent years. It has also been a way for me to vent my frustrations and the helplessness I have felt as I found myself without support. I'm sure that as more people learn about food allergies, their symptoms and what steps should be taken, many families will benefit.

I am not a doctor or nutritionist; I am the mother of children with allergies who for a long time did not know what was happening to my children, or how to help them. I want to share our story, along with the stories of other families with children with allergies, as a way to help more children receive a proper diagnosis and allow them to improve their quality of life.

A few years ago I found myself alone, angry, exhausted, with children who were sick all the time, and with no diagnosis. It was another family who, by sharing their story with me, gave me a clue to start investigating if my children could get better by assessing whether their illnesses were related to the food they ate. I believe that the experiences of others are very rewarding and can help us in our quest to describe a comprehensive clinical picture, with all the symptoms. This practice can give us ideas to explore the possibility that our children belong to the group of people whose bodies react in an exaggerated manner to a certain type of food, as if it were a bacteria or a virus, and therefore, are constantly sick and with weakened systems that cause chronic diseases.

In most cases, doctors focus only on the symptoms, which in these cases are varied and particular to each person, ranging from diarrhea, vomiting, and rhinitis to frequent colds, just to name a few. My journey with doctors was long, frustrating, and difficult because, despite trying various treatments and visiting doctors with various specialties, I did not get favorable results; things only got worse. My children had diverse symptoms that specialists related to a single cause, and were treated with drugs that only treated the symptoms. This, coupled with frequent fevers, caused them to be weak, underweight and with weak immune systems.

Because creating a diagnosis for them is difficult, many sick children, and adults as well, for whom these symptoms have become chronic and a part of their daily life, take medication to help them overcome the crisis, and they are simply accustomed to not feeling well most of the time. I include myself in that group.

In this search, I realized that we have forgotten our intuition: as mothers we know that something is wrong, that the doctor has not made the right diagnosis, that the child is reacting poorly to the medication or maybe that we should go to another doctor. But often we do not listen to ourselves and we have to remember that, as parents, we are the ones who know our children best and know what is normal and what is not, what they eat, how they sleep, how they behave, so we can suspect that something is wrong.

It's also my dream, that this book can offer support for those currently living with allergies, and who are in constant search for new food choices. Additionally, I want to inform those who are unfamiliar with this subject so that they may understand and respect when a person suffers from these conditions and must follow a special diet. Not everyone tolerates food in the same way, and what is delicious and nutritious for some may be harmful to others.

In recent years I have met other families in the same situation and exchanged ideas, suggestions, and recommendations to make this experience more bearable. I have also found solidarity and understanding, as well as appreciation from many people.

The lack of information to achieve the proper diagnosis is one of the main problems and obstacles. This book addresses this issue from a practical, simple, and concrete standpoint in order to facilitate decision-making regarding the care of our health.

Does your child have flu-like symptoms throughout the year? Do they cough constantly? Is your child often constipated? Do they have problems in their sleeping habits? Do they have unexplained diarrhea? Do they complain of recurrent stomachaches? Is your child below the average height and weight of children their age? Have you consulted with several doctors and, despite following the treatment, your child remains sick? If the answer is yes, read on and discover the answer to the greatest of all questions: What to do about it?

This book does not replace the diagnosis of a medical specialist. The opinions given here are personal and based on experience.

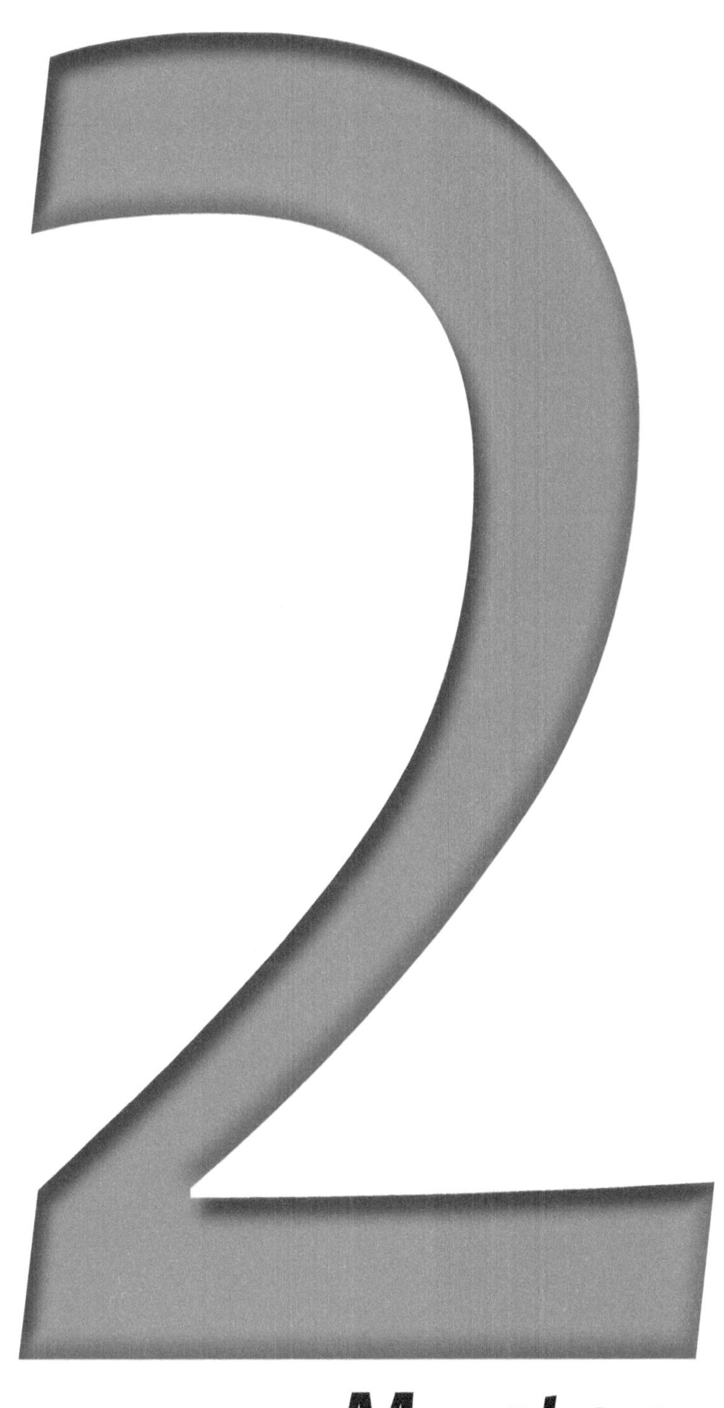

My story

a. Habits

I come from a family of nine children; three of my siblings had severe allergies throughout childhood. It was the early eighties, and what they recommended to people with this condition were long periods of vaccines, which are applied in the arm once or twice a week. My brother Peter also developed asthma during his childhood; he suffered several major attacks requiring hospitalization. The word allergy is a term familiar to me since childhood.

Of the twenty-three grandchildren in my family, 45% have been diagnosed with a condition related to allergies. Some had to undergo adenoid operations and had to have tubes in their ears; others were hospitalized with severe gastrointestinal disorders; only seven were diagnosed correctly when younger: the discomfort was caused by food. I had never given much importance to my family history until now, when I found a common denominator: genetics and food, a trigger for discomfort.

I grew up with a diet rich in dairy; the basics for me were milk, cheese, and yogurt, not to mention ice cream. I ate everything and overall I felt healthy, although with some digestive disorders that I believed to be hereditary or due to stress. Now I know the real cause.

b. The Battle Begins

b.1 The Physical Side

It was with Alejandra, my eldest daughter, that I began this journey. She was a very healthy baby; I breastfeed her for nine months. The introduction of solid foods was just as the doctor recommended. She did not tolerate formula, as it caused constipation and an upset stomach, so after weaning we fed her with soy milk, and she tolerated it without problems. She was a very healthy girl, until she was two years old. In January 2003, Alejandra began to attend day care and at the same time she began to get sick frequently. That is when a battle against a seemingly invisible and undetectable disease first began.

She got sick twice a month. Sometimes there were only bouts of fever lasting from forty-eight to seventy-two hours and as soon as the symptoms began, they disappeared. Dr. "X", our pediatrician, would prescribe medicines for fever, such as acetaminophen or ibuprofen, but she often had respiratory complications. She was coughing constantly. My husband and I spent many sleepless nights, as we took turns caring for her because her coughing was very intense and frequent; she couldn't go three minutes without coughing, so we gave her water, medicine, suppositories. One night my husband even sat her by his side to sleep in that position, and still she spent the whole night coughing every three minutes. In search of options that would soothe the cough, I turned to thyme cream, eucalyptus spray, and any home remedy that was recommended to me to try to relieve her coughing. We tried many things out of desperation. The mucus never stopped, she had a runny nose all the time, and this often complicated the state of her breathing passages. On top of all of this, we had to give her antibiotics.

I remember two episodes of vomiting that lasted all

night. I took her to my bed; I slept with a pot next to me because we couldn't make it to the bathroom. I had to watch her closely since, even though she didn't have anything in her stomach, she kept vomiting up water and gastric juices. The next day, I took her for a check-up with her pediatrician who sent her to undergo a variety of tests; the results were normal. There seemed to be no explanation for the symptoms.

Alejandra had a large appetite, but remained underweight. On three occasions I had to take her to the emergency room for vomiting and diarrhea. When she had new tests as ordered by the pediatrician, the results were again normal. The diagnosis, in the words of the doctors, was "a virus". We did tests for rotavirus more than four times, and they all came back negative. I realized that a "virus" in the stomach and respiratory tract was constantly attacking my daughter. What's happening? It's nothing? I do not understand, we go to the best doctors, we try many options and nothing makes it better, someone please help me! Is it normal? Are we exaggerating as first-time parents? What was certain is that not having a good night's sleep was ruining our day.

In March 2005, my second child, Patricio, was born. He was also fed with breast milk. He was a baby who often suffered from colic. The pediatrician prescribed medication for colic for four months. For my part, I still had a diet rich in dairy products. At that time I knew it was important to look after my diet, as any substance that I ate passed to him through my milk, but I never suspected that the cow's milk I consumed had to do with his cramps. It was not until I started giving him formula that Patricio began to have a fever regularly and constant rhinitis, even with soy milk.

Something was wrong: my two children were sick all the time. One got sick one weekend and the other the next. They were normally getting sick in three-week cycles and the unexplained fever returned. I woke up frequently during the night to take their temperature, give them medicine or bathe them, as well as deal with the persistent cough. My husband and I wondered what kind of weekend we would have, a sick one or a normal one.

Doctors would prescribe antibiotics, but only two weeks would pass and they would get sick again with a fever, or ear, or throat infections.

I felt misunderstood, lonely, anxious, bewildered. I went to the best doctors, followed all medical instructions, cared for them as best as I could, and they just got worse, especially Alejandra, who by then was four. She loved milk, ate large quantities of all kinds of cheeses, yogurts for children, etc.

Every time I went to the pediatrician I asked for some explanation of why they both got sick, especially her. His answer was that by attending school, she was contracting some viruses, and that Patricio was contracting them from his sister. I understand they occasionally contract them once in a while, like other children, but this was more than average; it was not normal. I compared them with children from their school and it was very noticeable that Alejandra was sick at least once a month.

In one of the many visits to Dr. "X", I insisted I wanted to take Alejandra to be evaluated by an allergist and, without much interest, he agreed. However, he said the following in an annoyed tone:

"But I'm sure it's not allergies. You're wrong. I do not know where you got this idea."

I went with a highly regarded allergist, Dr. "Y", who performed the allergy skin test (Appendix 2). This test involves placing needles on the patient's back with substances such as caffeine, strawberry, and some pollen, among others. If after a period of five to ten minutes of exposure a rash appears, it indicates that the patient is allergic to that substance. In the case of Alejandra, everything was negative, except for a slight allergy to caffeine. Doctor "Y" recommended that I stop giving her chocolate and coffee (which she did not drink anyway) as well as treatment with bacterial vaccines that would help improve her immune system. The treatment lasted six months and she was given one vaccine per week during this time. After paying for this expensive treatment, plus six months of visits and consultations, Alejandra's health remained the same. I felt embarrassed, I was sure that the specialist would have the answers to my questions and, after six months, I was still confused, enduring my children's crises.

That was when I decided to visit another pediatrician that we knew, Dr. "A", to ask his opinion. He recommended taking Alejandra to an immunologist to evaluate and verify that she does not suffer from an immune system disorder. I went immediately to Dr. "B", who requested blood tests of all immunoglobulins to rule out insufficiency in the immune system that could be compromising her health. Silently, I prayed for this specialist to finally give me a logical explanation. I prayed that the tests they were going to perform on my daughter would provide some answers, so that she could be treated and my children could improve their health even in the slightest. The test results were normal, indicating that her immune system was working perfectly. Honestly, I was surprised! I was sure something would appear; some clue that would allow me to find an answer. Now where would I go? What specialist should be consulted? What more could I do for my children? Dr. "B" only said that Alejandra was within the range considered normal and gave me no further recommendations. I, who cared for and lived with the girl around the clock, knew something was not right. However, at that time I had no idea what else to do to help her and get a compelling and definitive diagnosis. I visited a homeopathic specialist, who said he could help, but his treatment did not work either.

There was also the economic aspect: paying for medical bills, lab tests, and treatments was a great expenditure for my family. My house was more like a pharmacy with the amount and variety of drugs that were in it. Our family dynamics were affected because we almost always had a sick child to care for, and our stress just increased.

b.2 The Emotional Side

One day my sister asked me:

"Could it be that you make them sick? You get hysterical every time your children are ill. Maybe you transmit your anger, your emotions to them."

It was true! Every time one of them began to have a fever, or just hearing them cough, I got angry and it caused me stress, because I knew I was still immersed in a seemingly endless cycle. I broke down and cried easily and was anxious most of the time.

Other people who wanted to support and encourage me would say:

"When they turn five, they will not get sick anymore."

"That's how children grow up, sick. It will pass."

"Why do you care so much about the flu?"

"But she looks great. Your daughter is so happy and nice."

Few knew of the long, sleepless nights, weekends locked away, the parties and school days she missed, and the number of doctor visits and trips to the pharmacies.

And then, the guilt washed over me. I constantly asked myself: What did I do wrong? Did I not dress them warm enough? Have I forgotten some medical advice? How did they become infected? I feared that, because of something I did wrong, I had caused their relapses. Since I was responsible for their care, who else could be the culprit?

Mainly my family, with all the love and intention to help, showered me with recommendations on how to cover them as they got out of the bath, to put warm clothes on them. “But it’s summer!” I said to myself.

I went to therapy to see if I was the problem. I was willing to work on myself in all that was necessary if that could help the children. However, deep down my inner voice told me I was not the problem. At that time, I was in school for my second degree in human development and until then I had worked hard on myself, my past and everything in my life that was still unresolved. I understood the close relationship mothers have with their children and that we are able, unconsciously, to affect them with our outstanding issues. I read several books and performed various exercises and, although this was a great help and relief, it did not rid the children of their mucus and fevers. The guilt made me feel worse. It was a burden for me to carry, and it filled me with anxiety and stress. I was also very angry with the doctors. We had visited several, and they had given my children many drugs and they always relapsed. It was nothing personal, but I went to several specialists and the situation never changed: there were no answers, no results. I felt exhausted and the children got weaker and weaker.

My husband was very concerned: helping me constantly with changing sheets and pajamas, bathing the children at midnight, giving them medicine, accompanying them as they struggled to sleep. It made me feel like I was not alone, and although it was a difficult time for the family, he always said that we would come out ahead. His optimism and hope kept us strong during those years.

c.3 The Hopeful Side

I still remember the day in January 2006 when Angel, a family friend, came to our house for a get-together. We had not seen each other in a long time, but he told us about his children and his new diet. I had no idea why he was telling us all this, but I listened carefully.

His son David was diagnosed with autism because he had some symptoms of the disorder, such as isolation and language delay. The psychiatrist they consulted with prescribed medication for him. The boy also had chronic constipation, sleep disorders and stomach problems. When he turned five, they took him to see a clinical dietician who, after performing blood tests to detect allergies and heavy metals, diagnosed him with food allergies: wheat, dairy and eggs. By changing his diet and starting dietary supplements, his recovery had been very favorable. The constipation he had suffered since he was a baby was gone. They completely stopped giving him the drug prescribed by the psychiatrist, and he continued improving drastically. He started speech therapy, and now David is a healthy young boy and continues with his diet, along with his entire family.

After listening to his story, I asked him for the phone number of his physician with the feeling that maybe he could help my children. No one had told me that food could compromise health to that extent before. We had already tried all the drugs and vaccines available. It was time to test a new theory.

Dr. "C", a physician specializing in clinical nutrition, received me warmly. He asked me a lot of questions, but above all he wanted to know what we ate. I explained the long list of symptoms and diseases that my children had. He immediately suggested a change in diet, consisting of completely eliminating milk and wheat, while at the same time requesting blood tests to identify food allergies. The test included a long list of ninety foods from different types of meats, fruits and vegetables, eggs, nuts, and cereals, which he would review to determine the level of allergy to each.

He also prescribed vitamins and supplements to help my children feel better and strengthen their immune system, but the biggest change came when we started the diet. The results of the blood tests surprised me: my daughter was suffering from a severe allergy to eggs, bananas, and, with less intensity, chocolate, nuts, almonds, milk, and yellow dye. She consumed large amounts of the types of foods for which resulted with a higher level of allergy in the test results. Patricio, being younger and having less time to eat a wider variety of foods, presented lower levels of allergy, but they were still important to give me clues about the ones that might cause problems, such as milk, beans, chocolate, nuts, and almonds.

So, in February 2006, my children began a strict diet. I went to the kitchen and emptied the pantry and refrigerator of all the foods they could not eat. I focused on everything they could eat, and I personally started to prepare their food to know precisely what they were eating. I began to notice many changes almost immediately: the rhinitis (runny nose or congestion) and chronic cough disappeared. It was a great pleasure to see that Alejandra was not congested and that the cough had disappeared; I could almost see a glimmer of hope. However, her fever continued to appear along with frequent bouts of tonsillitis, so it was necessary to have surgery to remove them the same year. Shortly after, between the diet and the tonsillectomy, my daughter's life changed; she gained over ten pounds in one year and did not have fevers, vomiting, coughing, or congestion. One day she approached me, looked me in the eye and with a tender smile on her face told me:

"Hey Mom, I haven't been sick in a long time."

Indeed, it had been more than six months without her getting sick.

I remember the summer of 2006, when Patricio was fifteen months old, he started having problems sleeping. For three months he would wake up every night, as if it was daytime; he played, talked, and took up to two hours to get back to sleep. Since he had already began the diet, I had become more observant. After many sleepless nights and analyzing what might be altering it, I thought it might be the banana because Alejandra had been diagnosed with a severe allergy to this fruit. Moreover, I had heard of the case of Rebeca, a three-year-old girl who had occasional behavioral problems caused by the high lithium content of bananas. Patricio loved bananas; he ate one or two a day. I decided to see what would happen if we stopped giving them to him, and that was the solution. From the day I removed them from his diet, Patricio went back to sleep all night and bananas disappeared forever from my house.

In November 2006, he had a relapse from eating

green beans, and in my ignorance, I still included them in his diet. It was complicated as he had serious ear infections for four consecutive months, during which he was prescribed various antibiotics. But since he continued to eat green beans, he would relapse and start all over again, to the extent that, in March 2007, he needed tubes in his ears to relieve the fluid buildup in them, which cured him completely.

My son significantly improved his language, which had not been very clear for a child his age, as well as his conduct and sleep. Patricio was usually irritable and often awoke at night crying and kicking.

Today I can recognize when Alejandra and Patricio eat something that is harmful for them because both immediately start with a cough or rhinitis. When this happens, my pediatrician has instructed me to administer oral medication for allergies (desloratadine or loratadine), which helps stop the allergic process.

Because we moms easily forget the moments of extreme tiredness and stress, I have no idea how many times I had to take them to a doctor on a weekend, or how long they took antihistamines, or the nights of poor sleep from coughing or fevers. The pediatrician, Dr. "X", who was my children's doctor during this time, for reasons I do not know and his apparent lack of ethics, would not provide my children's records to refresh my memory when writing this book. I was very bothered by his attitude, his apathy, and his nonsensical explanations. He told me I should have asked when I changed doctors. I believe the real reason is he recognizes he could not handle the case.

I notified him at the time that my children's problems had been food allergies, including milk, to which Dr. "X" responded again that he did not think that would have been the cause of their frequent illnesses. Doctor "Y" just kept silent.

C. Drastic Changes

Once I had the results in my hand, and as I carefully watched what foods each child ate, we began a new stage in the life of our family. We cleaned out our pantry and refrigerator, leaving out the dairy (milk, all kinds of cheeses, yogurt, cream), wheat (pasta, breads, cereals, tortillas, flour, biscuits), eggs, bananas, chocolate, beans, zucchini, tomatoes, walnuts, almonds, artificial colors and additives.

Our diet was very healthy, with chicken, meat, fish, corn and rice, chickpeas, lentils, beans, and fruits and vegetables, except those mentioned above.

I confess that this new diet was difficult to do, especially since, in order to avoid any mistakes, I had to prepare all meals to know exactly what my children were eating. Much of the success was based on symptoms or observing whether there were changes after eating a meal; in order to determine which food had caused it. Blood tests were performed to diagnose them; however, they were inconclusive. The blood work only showed what foods had caused a chronic injury, so I had to discover the other foods that still caused them discomfort.

One practice that I started doing was to carefully review the ingredients of any prepared foods I bought to see if the children could eat them. I still do, mostly because they do not tolerate the dyes, preservatives, nuts, and almonds contained in cookies and cereals.

Each time I left the house, I had to bring their food to make sure what they ate did not hurt them. At home, we all tried to adapt and be supportive of each other; so my husband and I did not eat what they did not eat, so it was easier to maintain the new diet.

Our kids have been great teachers for us through their discipline and self-control. They have understood the great benefits of following the plan; they understood and respected it, and they noticed that they felt healthier and want to continue feeling this way. But those who did not understand were the people around us – family and friends – who often questioned our habits. They did not understand that the diet was not a whim or a fad, but that, in truth, the children got sick when they were given meals outside their diet. School and children's parties became a challenge, since I had to call ahead or bring our own snacks to avoid problems.

I felt alone in the process, but when I saw my children with more stable health, I had no doubt that we were on the right track and it was worth the effort. I always had the support of my husband, who supported me from the beginning, and as he saw the changes in the children, he also understood the importance of the diet.

When I was pregnant with our third child, I cut out dairy completely, on the recommendation of Dr. "C", with the hope that it would reduce the chances that the baby was allergic. During pregnancy and nursing, I noticed that it improved my health by reducing the frequency of my allergic rhinitis, my constant vaginal discharge and infections, and my bowel distension disappeared. It even took away the dark circles under my eyes. Even when I finished nursing, I realized that I felt much better without dairy and, if I mistakenly had some, I was terribly sick to my stomach or would end up with a respiratory or vaginal infection. My husband also decided to eliminate dairy products from his diet and found that his dark circles, the small constant cough, recurrent colds, and constipation disappeared.

We became more observant and noticed how some other types of food produced other symptoms; for instance, walnuts led to bloody stools, and vinegar and beans to diarrhea. We realized that we constantly lived with these symptoms, and we had become used to living like this. By making a radical change in our diet, we saw how good we felt. We eliminated some things and replaced them with others; for example, instead of cereal with milk in the morning we would have egg whites with turkey breast, or instead of quesadillas at dinner we would have a tuna salad. There are foods that did not return to my kitchen: box cereals (containing many dyes and preservatives), packaged cookies and crackers (except the simplest, such as salted crackers), and of course any dairy (including ice cream, pizza, etc.) I started to modify and invent recipes and began substituting some ingredients for others in our favorite recipes, ensuring that they were very tasty and the kids loved them.

I became more aware of what we ate, trying not to buy prepared foods or frozen or processed foods, and to identify the ingredients they contain more easily. I got used to reading labels and asking what is in the dishes we are being served wherever we go. Some friends began to understand our new way of eating and now even prepare special dairy-free desserts for us.

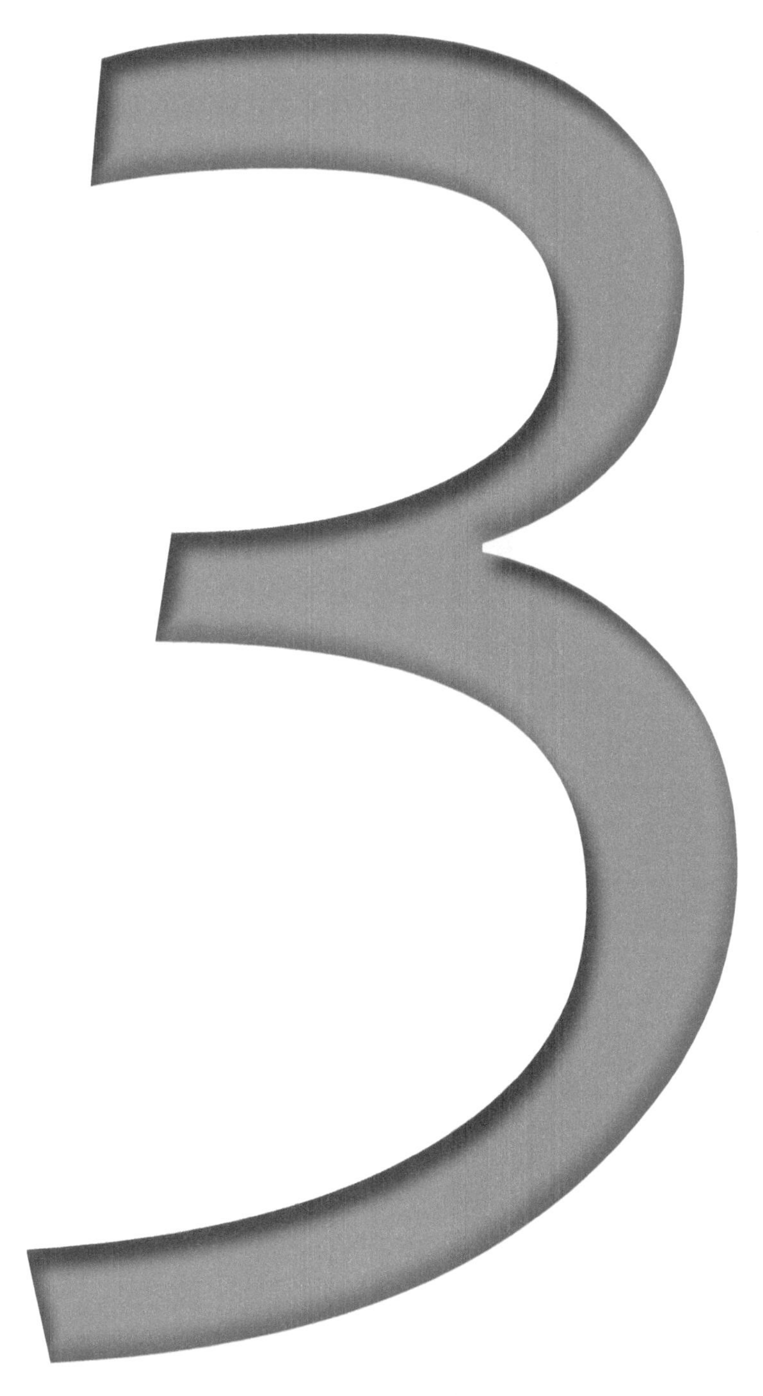

Food Allergies

a. What are they? What are the Symptoms?

I'd like to share some of what I learned on this subject; to show what we are talking about, and thus have more tools to know what to do and with whom to work.

In the United States, today more than 12 million people suffer from food allergies, equivalent to four percent of the population of the country; about 3 million are children. The incidence is higher in children under the age of three[1]. In a study conducted in Mexico City, of a group of 4,742 people aged 0 to 98, 42.6% had two or more allergy symptoms, and 20% of those with allergies were younger than six[2].

The Mexican Association of Pediatrics (Asociación Mexicana de Pediatría) defines a food allergy as "an immune reaction resulting from the consumption of a food," while food intolerance is "the abnormal response to a food or food additive that occurs in some individuals, in which an immune mechanism has not been demonstrated".[3] In addition, Kathleen Mahan, author of the book Krause's Food, Nutrition, & Diet Therapy, adds that in order for a reaction to a food allergy to exist, the gastrointestinal tract needs to absorb proteins and other large food molecules that interact with the immune system and generate a response. In normal situations, the gastrointestinal tract and system raise a barrier that prevents the absorption of almost all intact proteins. When the barrier is crossed, an allergic sensitization may occur, and re-exposure triggers an allergic reaction.[4] Mahan continues by asserting that immunoglobulins play a significant role in food allergies. The types of immunoglobulins include IgG, IgM, IgD,

IgA, and IgE – the latter is responsible for handling the predisposition to allergic reactions.

The prevalence in children is variable. According to different studies, it ranges from 0.3% to 12%. In adulthood, this range is 3% to 4%.[5] On the other hand, there is a higher percentage of intolerance or sensitivity; up to 13.5% of the population suffers from one.[6]

The range of symptoms that are usually present is very diverse, so it is important to mention them and realize that they affect each individual differently. They can occur immediately after eating the food, after a short time period ranging from 2 to 24 hours (Type 1), or later, after 24 hours (Type 3). They occur most frequently in the gastrointestinal tract, on the skin, or in the respiratory system.

In an interview, Dr. Gerardo Velazquez, a pediatrician with expertise in clinical nutrition, shared his definition with me:

The issue of food allergy or hypersensitivity is very complex and has been studied from many perspectives. There is literature based on anecdotes and literature based on scientific rigor. Not all the information available has the support of evidence-based medicine. It is important to distinguish between "allergy or hypersensitivity" and food intolerance. I'll explain:

A) Food Intolerance: *Although there are intolerances to many other foods, the best known classic intolerance is that of lactose, which is the carbohydrate in milk. This term is directly related to a lack of maturation of the* *digestive processes; for example, lactase, which is the enzyme responsible for digesting lactose, is produced in the fetus beginning in weeks 32-34 of pregnancy, but it is not until the child is three or four years old that the amount and quality of the enzyme is adequate. For this reason many children are lactose "intolerant" when they are young and can later tolerate this type of food. In the same way, it is believed that the lactase producing gene is modified by the environment, and the act of putting the patient into contact with dairy products, especially milk, will finally stimulate the establishment of production. In this sense, there are three types of patients with lactose intolerance:* **1) Ethnic intolerance:** *the most frequent, it is believed that over 70% of the population older than 25 years of age do not tolerate milk and dairy products.* **2) Secondary intolerance:** *this is very frequent in babies with gastrointestinal infections, especially viruses such as rotavirus. Ideally, lactose must be eliminated for two to four weeks while the intestinal inflammation subsides, and later on the child will tolerate dairy again.* **3) Congenital lactose intolerance:** *these patients are very rare. This is the classic patient who is never able to tolerate dairy and should be fed with "milk" that does not originate from animals: soy, almond, etc.*

Typical symptoms are bloating (gas), abdominal distension, occasional reflux, diarrhea, cramps. But there are usually no systemic reactions such as rhinorrhea, dermatitis, eczema, asthma, or anaphylaxis.

B) Food Allergy or Hypersensivity: *It is accepted that there are "classical allergenic" foods such as cow's milk, eggs, soy, wheat, and different types of nuts like peanuts, walnuts, almonds, etc. These foods may also cause the symp-*

toms described above, but there are also other symptoms that suggest that the problem has to do with hypersensitivity, such as runny nose, eczema, dermatitis, asthma, and anaphylaxis. There was even one patient who had a fever after eating a pear. The symptoms can be very specific, like that of one of my children who is allergic to peaches, but they may also be allergic to gluten. In this case, the number and variety of foods that trigger the reaction is very broad: noodles, bread, cookies, and anything containing wheat. This includes foods not referred to as classic sources of gluten, such as food preservatives containing glutamate, which is a derivative of gluten.

As described by Dr. Velasquez, the symptoms are often very different, so it is important to know them and verify whether they can be associated with an allergy.

Symptoms of Food Allergy According to Mahan [7].

Gastrointestinal:

- Abdominal pain
- Nausea
- Vomiting
- Diarrhea
- Gastrointestinal bleeding
- Protein-losing enteropathy

- Itching in the mouth and throat

Skin:

- Urticaria (Hives)
- Eczema
- Angioedema
- Erythema
- Pruritus (Itching)

Respiratory Tract:

- Rhinitis
- Asthma
- Cough
- Heiner syndrome (milk-induced respiratory attack)

Systemic:

- Anaphylaxis

Controversial and Unsubstantiated:

- Behavioral conditions

- Strain and fatigue syndrome
- Attention Deficit Disorder
- Otitis media
- Psychiatric disorders
- Neurological symptoms
- Musculo-skeletal alterations
- Migraine headache

There are other symptoms mentioned by other authors, and it seems important to mention them because, although it has not been proven, it has been found that they may be related to allergies. In my experience, I identified many of them in my own case and in other experiences. Among the symptoms mentioned are: disturbed sleep, waking up early in the morning unable to return to sleep, recurrent ear infections, abdominal pain, swelling after eating, gas, autism, vaginal discharge, and aggressive or irritable behavior,[8] as well as colitis, constipation, sinusitis, myalgia, fever, and enuresis.[9] Others, which are still under debate, are prolonged fever, nephrotic syndrome, seizures, headache, arthritis, vasculitis, fibromyalgia, thrombocytopenia, and constipation, among others.[10]

There are also different hypersensitivity reactions:

Type I or immediate: genetic predisposition that will

develop the production of IgE specific to the food, with consistent symptoms (urticaria, angioedema, and anaphylaxis) with re-exposure to the food.

Type II or antibody-dependent cell-mediated cytotoxicity: mostly exhibited as anemia, leukopenia, and thrombocytopenia.

Type III or immune complex: evident as fever, lymphadenopathy, rash, vasculitis, and proteinuria.

Type IV or cellular involving T lymphocytes: mechanism involved in gastroenteropathy and contact dermatitis.

The most frequent presentation is the type I reaction, followed by a mixed presentation (one or more mechanisms involved in one patient), which are followed by types IV, III, and II, respectively.[11]

Although allergens can be found in many foods, 90% come from the proteins found in milk, eggs, seafood, nuts, peanuts, soybeans, and wheat. Some additives can also cause allergic responses, especially those contained in preservatives.[12] There is another important food group, including: sesame, sunflower, cotton and poppy seeds, beans, tartrazine (yellow dye 5), sulfites (found in preservatives) and latex, which, along with the first eight, make up 95% of the causes of food allergies.[13]

Most doctors usually treat isolated symptoms, prescribing medication to control them; never knowing what causes them, and that is where we get lost, just covering what the body is saying to us through various manifestations. We silence it and saturate it with drugs and antibiotics, and this can last for years before anyone suspects that something is wrong.

Now, it is important to note that there are other types of allergies:

1. *By Contact:* produced by touching the skin to the allergen, which may be a plant, jewelery, latex, or a beauty product.

2. *Injectable:* insect bites, animal bites, medication.

3. *Inhaled:* pollens, animal dander, dust mites, spores, cigarette smoke, chemicals.[14]

With so many symptoms, and their variations, the amount of food consumed, and since symptoms are so different for each individual, even within the same family, it is very difficult to reach a definitive diagnosis or definition of a food allergy or intolerance. Usually the doctor will be interested in curing the symptoms without questioning or inquiring about the origin of the disease. Although often they are the result of common bacterial or viral infections in childhood, when symptoms are recurring, or even when you have followed the treatment prescribed by your doctor, or taken long-term treatment and the child fails to improve, it gives us more clues as to believe that there may be an external factor that is making the child sick, whether it be what they eat, breathe, or touch.

b. Diagnosis

It is impossible to diagnose a food allergy in one test, as it requires a complete medical history and various studies.

This is where the difficulties begin for parents since, as I previously said, pediatricians usually treating symptoms as an isolated event. However, if we stack up a long list of visits, we must find a common denominator and start thinking whether there is any relation to food intake and the onset of symptoms.

Generally, diagnosis begins with an interview concerning the symptoms, what they are, when they started, a family history, and current diet. According to the American Academy of Allergy, Asthma and Immunology (AAAAI), if one parent has an allergy, the risk of the child suffering from allergies is 48%, and increases to 70% if both parents suffer from allergies.

Parents are often confused when giving a medical history because:

1. They attribute the symptoms to the last food that was ingested.

2. They believe their children have the same allergies as they do.

3. They tend to take the skin test results as conclusive and discard small symptoms.

4. They relate foods that the child does not like, believing that they are allergic to these foods, when they have little relation, according to Kumar.[15]

A good idea is to keep track of foods eaten and symptoms that occur, as it is difficult to remember everything. When notes are taken, parents can begin to associate symptoms with food.

Coupled with the history, there is some evidence that helps the doctor with the diagnosis, including skin tests and blood tests (RAST), which are verified once foods that test positive for allergies are removed and changes can be seen.

In addition to the removal of these foods, eliminating processed foods including breakfast cereals, cookies, and frozen or pre-prepared food is also recommended, as they contain many preservatives and dyes.

An elimination study can also be used, which consists of, for several weeks, removing foods that are suspected of causing the symptoms, then reintroducing them one by one, observing whether any symptoms appear. This can be a simple and effective test, though much depends on the removal of the right foods and making detailed observations. It is important to note that this process should be monitored by the specialist, in order to ensure that the child is well fed.

c. Treatment

Treatment for food allergies, after diagnosis, is very simple and is based on modifying the diet, eliminating foods that cause symptoms, allowing the body to regulate itself and get back into balance, which results in the person's health improving. It is an effective and safe procedure, if performed properly and for the amount of time necessary for the body to once again tolerate the food causing the allergy. The amount of time can be six months or a year for certain patients, while for others the new diet should be followed permanently, depending on the degree of sensitivity to that food.

We must also take care to see that the diet remains balanced, preferably supervised by a physician or nutritionist, so the child is well nourished and a variety of food is consumed. Give the child the opportunity to taste new foods that are not normally offered, that are very tasty, and have a high nutritional value such as lentils, chickpeas, pomegranates, soybeans, and oats.

It is also important to inform everyone in the household about their change in diet, to avoid confusion and a relapse.

There are several medications to reduce symptoms such as antihistamines, corticosteroids, and bronchodilators for the management of rhinitis, cough, and respiratory problems. In skin conditions, some specialized creams, and in cases of severe anaphylaxis, epinephrine injections can be used to stop acute reactions.[16] Always check with your doctor before you give any of these drugs to your children. There are also identification bracelets that indicate that the person is severely allergic to certain foods.[17]

People with food allergies have intestinal hyperpermeability, that is, their intestines allow large molecules to pass through their walls, causing allergies to occur. So it is important to help their body regenerate the intestine through dietary supplements and a special diet.

Several studies demonstrate the coexistence of different diseases with allergies in the same person. Ninety percent of asthma patients also suffer from allergic rhinitis.[18] Allergic rhinitis affects the sufferer's social life, sleep, school, and work. Its economic impact is considerable, although it is still under-diagnosed and under-treated. It is estimated that over 600 million patients worldwide suffer from it.[19] According to a study conducted by surveying parents of asthmatic children in the city of Monterrey, Nuevo León, Mexico, they spend, on average, $225 annually on consultations, $134 on immunotherapy, $45 on emergency room visits, and $180 on hospitalizations.[20]

A study was conducted involving migraine sufferers concerning the presence of IgG antibodies against food. The treatment they were given was to remove from their diet the foods that tested positive in the study, which then controlled the migraines without the need for medication.[21]

As I previously said, I did not have sufficient advice and support from my previous pediatrician to know it was time for my children to be evaluated by a specialist. Because of that, I had no way to know that their recurring illnesses indicated of something more that should be reviewed. In my search, I found the following recommendations.

According to the AAAAI, an evaluation should be done by a specialist in the following circumstances:

* Chronic or recurrent infectious rhinosinusitis.

* Eight or more new infections in a year.

* Two or more severe unusual infections in a year.

* Two or more months of treatment with antibiotics, with little or no effect.

* Two or more cases of pneumonia within one year.

* A toddler who does not gain weight or grow normally.

* Recurrent abscesses within the skin or organs.

* Persistent fungal infection in the mouth or anywhere on the skin after the child's first year.

* Need for intravenous antibiotics to eliminate infections.

* Two or more infections of internal origin.

* Family history of immunodeficiency.

The American Academy of Pediatrics, meanwhile, proposes some considerations that may be effective for the prevention of allergies.

First, it proposes promoting breastfeeding, as breast milk has immunological capacity of immunomodulation and the development of bacterial flora that is essential for the development of allergies.

Second, adding foods after six months of age, with a specific delay in families susceptible to egg protein.

Third, in cases which require supplementation with formulas, giving preference to those with hydrolyzed or highly hydrolyzed cow's milk proteins.[23] As for soy milk, it has been shown that 3 to 10% of patients with an allergy to cow's milk proteins are also allergic to soy. A hypoallergenic diet for the breastfeeding mother (eggs, peanuts, fish) can also be considered, as they may pass food allergens through nursing and sensitize the infant.[24]

d. The 5 symbols allergies

+ MORE observation:

I think this is the focal point of this topic. I insist on it, and I encourage parents to become detectives, as they are the ones responsible for feeding their children. Parents should pay special attention to what their children consume. This closeness to them will allow parents to notice changes in their habits: appetite, behavior, sleep pattern. This also includes keeping track of illnesses, hospitalizations, and lab work, as well as diagnosis from every physician they have visited.

- LESS *waiting:*

If symptoms appear and, despite following the treatments prescribed by specialists, the child does not improve, or worsens, seek a specialist who has experience in managing food allergies and, if required, do skin or blood tests. Many children experience a significant positive change with the elimination of milk and some other food that is suspected to be related. Always monitor to ensure that the diet remains balanced.

× MULTIPLYING *effort:*

Once you have a diagnosis of food allergy, teamwork within the family will be critical to successfully implement and maintain the diet. Having at home only the food they can eat and adding new recipes to the family diet will enrich everyone's life. I even dare to say it will be a more nutritious and varied diet.

÷ DIVIDE *all foods:*

The choice of the variety of the diet will allow children to try foods that may be new to them, but that are no less tasty if prepared well. Parents play an important role as examples for their children: if mom and dad eat it, it will be a very natural invitation for children to follow suit.

∞ CONTINUE *evaluating:*

After the time period recommended by the specialist, reintroduce one food at a time to see if it will be tolerated; that is, when it is consumed, the child does not show any symptoms. Do this with every food. The waiting time varies from person to person. It is also likely that one food will have to be removed permanently.

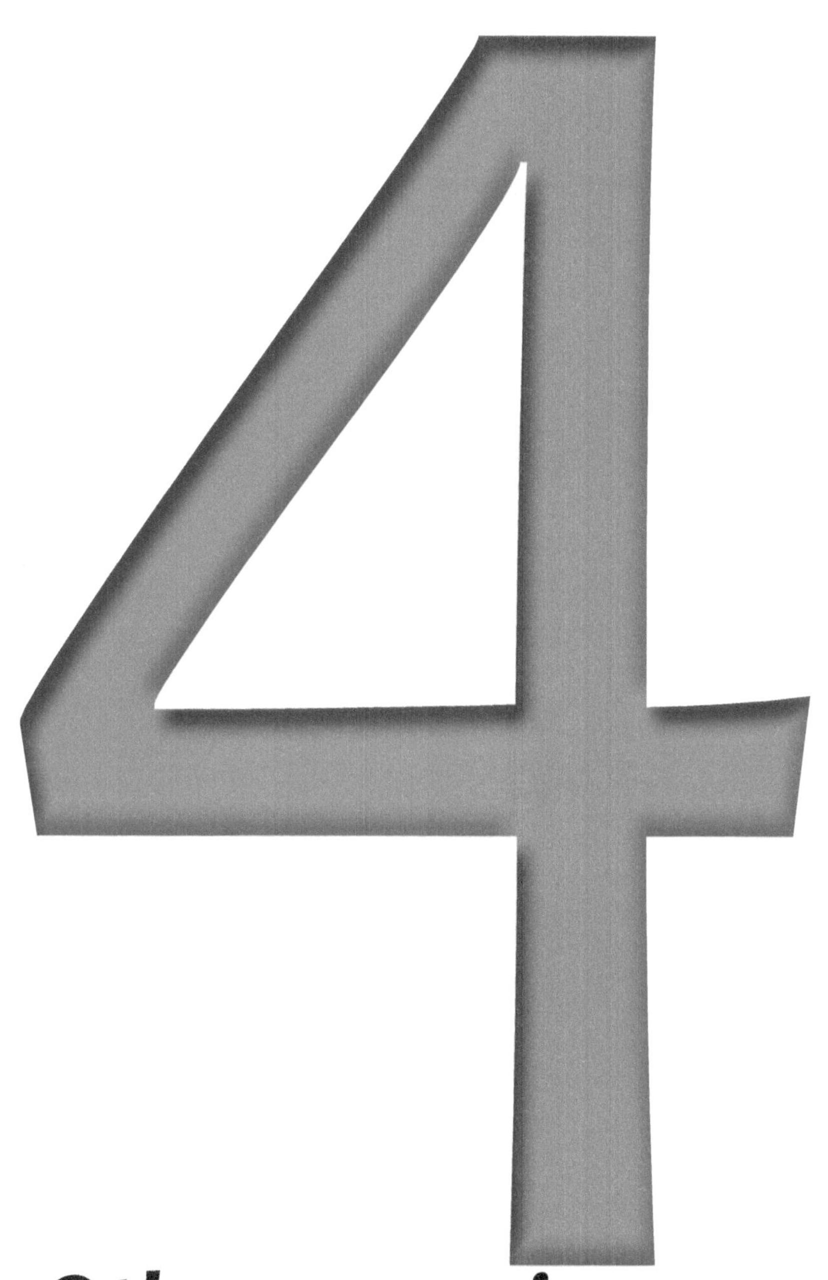

Other experiences

LUIS´ CASE

I have known Luis since he was born. His mother fed him milk and followed all the recommendations given by his pediatrician for the introduction of food. His father suffered from asthma as a child, and his health was compromised several times by asthma attacks, to the extent that he required hospitalization; so there is a significant genetic factor in this case. Luis began to show symptoms when eggs were introduced in his diet at the age of one. Ten minutes after being ingested, a strong allergic reaction began and his face, eyelids, and neck were covered with hives. The pediatrician prescribed an antihistamine, which managed to stop the allergic process. Luis was admitted to the hospital at two years of age due to severe diarrhea for prolonged periods without apparent cause, as well as rhinitis, which often ended in respiratory infections. He underwent an intestinal biopsy, along with other studies such as blood count and skin allergy tests, which were positive, mainly for strawberries, eggs, milk, spinach, and tomatoes.

Despite having a strict diet based on chicken, beef, rice, and some vegetables, the symptoms did not improve. His mother went through difficult times and could not find a diagnosis or cure for Luis; the constant diarrhea weakened him and affected his growth. I know she felt alone and misunderstood while searching day after day for something more to do to help her child. I did not know much about allergies at the time, and I confess that I did not understand; I thought she was exaggerating. I did not understand why she worried so much, and, for me, everything that happened to Luis was very rare. As his diet was limited, one day his mother sensed that perhaps the potatoes could be causing the diarrhea, so she removed them from his diet. And that was it! The potato was what caused the diarrhea, but it had not been discovered in any study. The discovery was the result of observation.

Luis was on a dairy-free diet until he was three, and was egg-free until the age of five. And even now, at ten, he tolerates many foods that before had caused him an allergic reaction. His mother is considering eliminating dairy again, as he often gets rhinitis and respiratory infections.[24]

Later, I experienced first-hand that same lack of understanding from other people who do not have sufficient information on the subject. That's why it's important to me that more people know what the families of those who are suffering from allergies go through. Loved ones are able to give the support these families need without judgment or criticism, but rather as a team to make the road a little easier.

ROBERTO´S journey

Roberto was born without any complications, and he was eighteen months old before the pediatrician noticed that he was below the normal weight and height for a child his age. At the age of two multiple antibiotics were prescribed, since he frequently had symptoms of throat infections and colds, which made the doctor think it might be a reason why the child was below the normal growth curve.

When he was two years and nine months old, he

fainted and fell unconscious for twenty minutes. At the hospital several tests were performed to determine what had happened, but none showed abnormal results. Roberto's parents were told that their son had a very high pain threshold, since on several occasions he showed no pain despite having injured a tooth or having bronchiolitis, so they had to be alert to any symptom, as it could be severe and the child probably would not show any reaction.

When Roberto was three, an endocrinologist diagnosed him with a growth hormone deficiency. A second diagnosis was insensitivity to the production of a growth hormone, although his body produced it, it was not being assimilated. The end result was that Roberto did not grow or gain weight.[25]

This was about the time when I met the boy. His mother was alarmed, since one of the alternatives was a drug therapy that, in addition to being expensive, had side effects. They did not know what to do or what the right decision was.

In recounting my experience, without being certain that Roberto's symptoms were due to allergies, his mother decided it was worth exploring the idea and rule out whether he had any food allergies.

They decided to have a specialist evaluate him and, after blood work and other tests to detect heavy metals, Roberto was found allergic to almost all the foods in the tests; among the highest were eggs, milk, salmon, beans, and soybeans. His mother stopped fixing food in aluminum pots and pans, which she replaced with stainless steel, since the small child's body had high concentrations of aluminum in it. Another doctor insisted that they follow a diet free of dairy, dyes, and preservatives.

With these adjustments, Roberto experienced a drastic change and, in the first month after implementing them, he grew four inches in height and gained two pounds in weight. It is important to remember that he had not gained any weight over the previous two years. However, their search did not end there, as he had to visit more specialists due to a condition in a heart valve. Roberto is now much better. Having spent more than a year on a strict diet, he is now stable, with slow but steady growth and no relapses.

Even though Roberto's case is complex, the change in his diet was a great improvement, which made it clear that everything matters, from the type of pots and pans in which we prepare food (which should be of stainless steel to avoid contaminating our food with heavy metals) to what we eat.

SINCE TWENTY-FIVE YEARS AGO

Although Daniel and Lucía are grown, their mother has not forgotten that they were allergic to milk and some other foods. She shared what happened to them twenty-five years ago: "When I changed Daniel from breast milk to formula at six months of age, he started getting diarrhea to the extent that we had to hospitalize him. Although doctors did not say anything to me, he was fed with soy milk in the hospital, which he tolerated well. I prepared all his baby food with fruits and vegetables, chicken, and rice. That's how I was able to help him move forward. When Lucía was born, I already had experience, and when she stopped drinking breast milk and formula was introduced and diarrhea began, I immediately knew she was allergic, too. Besides milk, they requested that I exclude from her diet eggs, chocolate, and strawberries. At six, she was a child who was often sick with throat problems and, when further tests were performed, we found that she was also allergic to beans.

Many times I despaired because I saw that my children did not grow at the same rate as other children. Currently my daughter is still very careful with what she eats; some foods such as milk, strawberries, and chocolate continue to cause troublesome symptoms, so she avoids them."[26]

Daniel and Lucía's mother found that the only way to ensure that her children did not eat something that hurt them was to prepare their food herself. Processed foods contain many ingredients, even in small doses, and when you want to avoid them, they are difficult to identify. In some countries, the labels where the ingredients are listed include in bold whether the product contains milk, nuts, eggs, wheat, or shellfish, which are the most common foods that cause allergies.

PABLO'S EXPERIENCE

Pablo began at the age of one to experience diarrhea and a frequent cough. He had these symptoms for one year. I met him during this time, as his mother was very concerned because the doctors had no idea what was causing this. They believed that it could be celiac disease, a condition in which the person is intolerant to gluten, which is contained mainly in wheat. An endoscopy was conducted and it confirmed that his intestinal villi was flattened. He was diagnosed with food malabsorption, so he started a very strict diet, mostly free of wheat, dairy, and eggs. His mother insisted he be evaluated to see if he had allergies. The doctor, somewhat reluctantly, agreed and referred him to an allergist. When the results came in, the recommendation was to eliminate twenty foods from his diet, in addition to following a special hygiene process to keep the boy free of dust and mites, as well as animal dander. By changing his diet, Pablo's improvement was noticeable; the symptoms disappeared completely. Many foods have now been reinstated to his diet without relapse.[27]

For Pablo's mother, it was clear that the diagnosis of food malabsorption was related to one of the symptoms, and she had to discover the real cause of her child's discomfort. She was the one who insisted that Pablo be assessed for allergies, but only months after the child began to be sick.

I insist that we seek answers! If what a doctor tells you does not answer all your questions, or if the treatment prescribed does not help, you should keep looking for a second, third, or fourth diagnosis until you find the solution.

JORGE'S changes

Jorge began to experience changes in his digestive system at the age of nine, characterized by bowel movements that were more frequent than usual. At the age of eleven he began to complain of severe pain in his lower abdomen, sometimes so intense that it pushed him to the point of tears, and he had bloody stools. His mother is a pediatrician and did not know what was wrong, so several tests were conducted: blood count, blood chemistry, liver function, and RAST (blood test for allergies). She consulted another doctor who recommended a diet free of milk and eggs. Since Jorge was already an older child, changing his diet was very difficult for him and his family, but when the diet was strictly followed, his symptoms decreased rapidly.

Three years later, his symptoms have disappeared and his health has been very good. Today, he is on a dairy-free diet.[28]

Children like Jorge, who understand when some types of foods are harming them and making them sick, take great interest in not eating that certain type of food. Of course, nobody wants to be sick on purpose; therefore, children become even more careful about what they eat and ask what is in the food before eating it. The symptoms are bothersome and can last several days, so they prefer to avoid them.

PAOLA'S story

Paola started with symptoms at the age of one. She was losing weight, not sleeping well or sleeping only a few hours during the night. She was irritable and suffered from constipation. Two years later she started to get sick every two weeks from fever and recurrent tonsil infections; she also had rhinitis constantly. Her mother and I talked at a meeting, or to put it a different way, we unburdened ourselves of what we were going through at that time, as our daughters are the same age. She decided to do allergy skin and blood tests, which were positive for various foods.

She began a diet and, although her mother noticed improvement, it wasn't until after her tonsils and adenoids were removed that her recovery was complete.[29]

To provide her with a greater variety of different types of food, Paola was given as meat rabbit, deer and quail. Variety is one of the secrets of success to eating a strict diet. There are different types of meat that can be included, as well as derivatives of corn and rice (pastas, milk, crackers). Nutritional rotation is important to avoid saturation of the body by the same food. Another option is to eat seasonal fruits, or to consume them during the months they are harvested and the following months to test the fruits of the corresponding seasons. Thus you rotate them all year, letting your body rest for several months.

WHEN I MET DIEGO AND ANDREA

I met them when they were three years old, but I knew nothing about their health until they were six years old, when I learned that Diego had been in the hospital and missed school for two months. It was then that I approached his mother to learn more about his history.

Diego and Andrea are twins, and starting at six months old they started to have recurrent ear and throat infections. At eight months they changed from formula to soy milk. Although Andrea improved after this change, Diego continued to have ear infections and required tubes in his ears and the removal of his adenoids. At eighteen months he relapsed, having throat infections with respiratory complications such as difficulty breathing and coughing fits. At the age of two, he was diagnosed with asthma and required the daily use of bronchodilators. Between the ages of two and five, Diego was in the hospital for pneumonia. At five he needed surgery to remove his tonsils and at six he was admitted for gastroenteritis. On that occasion he had to stay home for eight weeks because his immune system was very weak.

During these years, Diego was evaluated by several pediatricians, a pulmonologist, allergists, otolaryngologists and immunologists, as well as undergoing homeopathic treatment for a year and a half.

When I heard their story and I could see how weak Diego was, I told his mother our story. She decided to test whether her children might be suffering from the same problems as mine and, after just one visit to a specialist in clinical nutrition, she began a strict diet free of dairy and some other foods that she suspected could be the cause of symptoms, such as peanut butter and chocolate. The whole family started with the regimen and noticed immediate changes. For Andrea, she had apparent changes in behavior: her temper tantrums, moodiness, and nightmares disappeared. In Diego's case, the constant colds disappeared. Both gained weight and grew in height, their appetites improved, they slept better at night, and they showed improved hair growth.

His mother shared: "We went through many things. While the children were sick without knowing what it was that caused so many diseases, we faced economic, professional, and sentimental problems. When we explored the option that food allergies might be causing their symptoms, we were surprised because we put two and two together; this was the obvious answer and no doctor had been able to say it before."[30]

I confess. After seeing the drastic changes in Diego and Andrea, as well as in my children and the other experiences described here, combined with what I've learned in recent years, it has reinforced my need to share and report on this subject. Although much is known about it, when you are face to face with sick children, it is something that is not considered, nor is it diagnosed.

JENNIFER AND SAM´S story

When Jennifer and Sam's mother told me her story, I realized how complicated and severe neurological symptoms caused by food allergy can be. This is another family that after many years discovered the real cause of their children's symptoms. These children are now free of medications and a terrible diagnosis all thanks to a new diet.

I asked Jennifer and Sam's mom to share her story with the hope that it could help liberate families who are in their same situation and prevent other families from having to go through the same difficulties. Her son had autism and her daughter had extremely, horrible temper tantrums that would last for days.

"My husband and I cannot tolerate gluten, and a casein-free diet helps. My son was assessed by many doctors and therapists to have many indications of autism. At over three years old, he exhibited the development of a seven month old baby. We had him assessed before he began going to school, and decided to remove gluten and casein from his diet right before the school year. The teacher was puzzled as the assessment did not match the child; he was a true leader who followed directions. We slowly began to reintroduce a glass of milk with breakfast until we began getting calls from his teacher months later referring to his behaviorisms as being wild. After weeks of trying to figure out why he was fine at home and screaming at school, we removed the milk and got a call from his teacher that very day…"thank you, he's back to normal". Several times he has tried having milk regularly again and these attempts have resulted in diarrhea and severe stuttering. After implementing all the dietary adjustments and supplementing with ASD vitamins, several doctors and other professionals are surprised by our claim that he has autism. He is mainstreaming kindergarten this year.

My daughter has a different story. When I was diagnosed with celiac disease, she was two years old and had terrible diarrhea. We began the whole family on a gluten free diet and observed differences in their bodily functions. She ripped out her hair for several years and threw the most horrible temper tantrums. The only way we had to calm her was cold, cold showers. At midnight, this was often our last resort. After several doctors and psychiatrists, it was suggested when she was eight years old that she had severe food allergies. Her anxiety was too high to do traditional skin pricks, so my quest began to find a doctor who would draw her blood to test for IgG and IgE antibodies, which was quite the quest. We began using a facial soap on her, and within two days she had a rash on her. Finally, I had something to run with. I went down several chains of the company until I got to somebody who would research this soap to determine what food derivative was in it: corn. Before being able to run blood panels, suggestions were made to remove all toxins from the house, including pajamas. What could be in pajamas? The fire retardants in her pajamas made her feel like bugs and snakes were crawling all over her. Problem solved, she sleeps in her clothes. Once we had her allergy panel back, we found out she has a severe and immediate reaction to corn, delayed reactions to soy and all beans. So much for the vegetables my autistic son would eat: green beans and corn. They were removed from the house and improvements began. We now had her to a point that we could determine some other allergies. Through much reading and research, we determined tartrazine (a.k.a. yellow 5) and the vegetable (corn) glazed apples were the final adjustments needed. We found once we adjusted to pickles with turmeric, instead of yellow 5, and switched to organic apples that are not glazed with corn; she turned into the most lovable, calm, and hungry little girl.

My kids are label readers and loving it. We take our own drinks (homemade sodas) and ketchup to restaurants when we go. Due to celiac disease, we often cook at home anyway. We just had to tweak a few things and learn to make others...such as marshmallows and icing sugar. They all realize the necessities of the diet changes, as they see the horrors when a contamination is made."

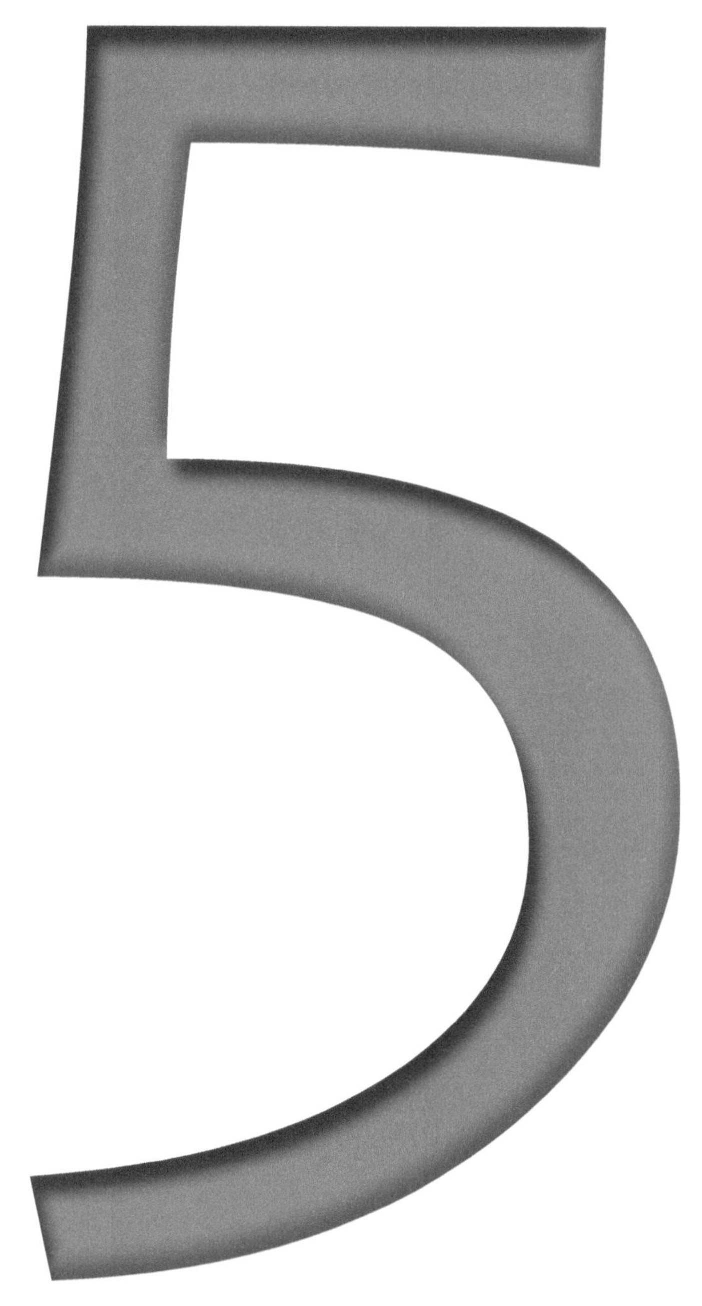

Myths and Customs

It is common for me to deal with questions and comments like:

"How do you avoid milk or cheese? Why?"

"But what do you feed your children if you do not eat all that?"

"Eat just a little; you'll see that you're OK."

"How do you it? I cannot live without milk."

"Aren't you overdoing it?"

I do not understand why people are so bothered that we do not consume milk. Is it an absolute reality that we cannot live without it? Is that the only food that exists in our diet? Lengthy discussions, even mockery, often erupt around this issue, especially in our inner circle, meaning family and friends.

At first, I spent a lot of time explaining what I discovered or read, but to no avail. It is difficult to understand when you're not living in the situation firsthand.

So I want to include some of what I have discovered about this food, milk, an ancient food, with strong cultural roots and highly overvalued. Throughout history, it has undergone significant changes, especially in the last hundred years, when technology has allowed it to be preserved for long periods of time and to be made into a host of other products. We are told that to be healthier, strong, and protected, we must consume it until old age; a belief that is becoming increasingly questionable.

Dr. Olga Cuevas, who has a PhD in biochemistry, is a dietary expert naturalist, and author of the classic book "The balance through food", published a nutritional and biochemical study of milk, in which she begins describing it as a "soup of proteins, hormones, fats, cholesterol, viruses, bacteria, and pesticides that can affect consumers in many ways".[31]

Let us start from the ground up: human milk is for human babies; it contains everything needed to feed and nourish them. Cow's milk is for calves, and its chemical composition is meant to nourish its own kind. So, as it is high in calcium, fat and phosphorus, it has a direct effect on the human body, mainly affecting the immune system.

Dr. Cuevas says that dairy products, given their high content of antigens, deplete the immune system, making the body more vulnerable to infections and diseases directly related to the system.

Several medical articles report that the human body itself, after infancy, decreases the production of lactase, the enzymes that digest lactose. This decline varies depending on the race and diet of the population concerned, but does not extend beyond the age of three.

A study done in 2007 showed that milk allergies may persist longer than previously thought. Out of 800 children suffering from milk allergies, only 19% had outgrown their allergy by the age of four and only 79% did at sixteen.[32]

One of the reactions of the organism is the excessive production of mucus, as a response mechanism of the immune system[33], often causing fluid to accumulate in the ears, sinuses, bronchi, and vagina, and, as time passes, the accumulation gives rise to infections, which will persist as long as the person continues to consume dairy.

It has been observed that there is an association of diabetes mellitus type I with an allergy to the proteins in cow's milk. The likely mechanism involved is the production of IgG antibody against bovine serum albumin, which cross-reacts with pancreatic beta cells and is manifested mainly in genetically predisposed individuals.[34]

Toxins, along with everything that the cow eats, are excreted through its milk. This means when we drink milk we also swallow pesticides, antibiotics, chemicals, and hormones, in addition to whatever the milk producers have added to create its derivatives such as cheeses and yogurts.

I believe it is important to mention that there are different types of reactions to cow's milk: lactose intolerance, allergies measured by IgE, and allergies not measured by IgE. In Table 1 we can see the main differences between them, in order to facilitate diagnosis and treatment.

Table 1. Differences between the different reactions to cow's milk [35]

	Lactose Intolerance	***Allergy through IgE***	***Allergy not through IgE***
Prevalence	High	Low	Low
Racial Variation	High	Low	Unknown
Common age	Adolescence / adulthood	Childhood	Childhood / adulthood
Cause	Lactose	Milk protein	Milk protein
Mechanism	Metabolic problem: low production of lactase	Immunological: IgE	Immunological: through cells, immune complex, other
Symptoms	Gastrointestinal	Gastrointestinal, skin, respiratory, anaphylaxis	Gastrointestinal and respiratory
Reaction time	0.5 - 2 hours	< 1 hour	> 1 hour or days
Tests	Lactose intolerance test, breath test, acid test, intestinal biopsy	Skin test and RAST	No simple diagnostic tests. Removal and testing
Prevention	Avoid lactose	Breastfeeding	Avoid consumption of milk protein

There is a misconception that we will not be well fed without milk and dairy products. Most people worry they will not consume enough calcium. However, contrary to popular belief, milk does not provide calcium due to its temporary acidity, which is caused by excess protein in dairy products and their high phosphorus content. This prevents the binding of calcium causing the body to lose more calcium than it gets, so it is not surprising that many people who consume high amounts of dairy have osteoporosis.

There are foods that are excellent sources of calcium. For example, almonds, hazelnuts, pistachios, sunflower seeds, broccoli, spinach, chard, olives, parsley, cabbage, soybeans, chickpeas, alfalfa sprouts, and spirulina are all high in calcium.[36]

Every day, more health specialists, especially those who work with alternative medicine such as homeopathy or Eastern medicine, gynecologists, oncologists and pediatricians recommend eliminating dairy from the diet, especially in patients complaining of skin allergies, respiratory, stomach, diabetes, cancer and hormonal problems, among others.

Did you know that the pasteurization of milk destroys vitamins and enzymes necessary for digestion? All the processes that it has to pass through in order to eliminate bacteria and microorganisms, as well as to improve its flavor and texture, makes it more difficult to absorb and affects the intestine because it cannot digest it properly, which may trigger many diseases such as chronic fatigue and various intestinal disorders.

Dr. Robert Cohen, author of several books, including "Milk A-Z" and "Milk, The Deadly Poison", explains at length the diseases associated with the consumption of milk, from allergies, to various types of cancer, to multiple sclerosis.[37] In the book Your Life in Your Hands, Dr. Jane Plant, tells how she recovered from breast cancer. She made important discoveries about how food is related to cancer. After surgery and other treatments such as chemotherapy and radiation therapy, the doctors were unable to control the progression and recurrence. She made important changes in her diet, eliminating dairy and other foods, thus completely eradicating the cancer that afflicted her.

She adds that in China, one in ten thousand women die from breast cancer, unlike in the U.K., where one in twelve women die of the disease, and in other Western countries the figure continues to rise to one in ten. She discovered that genetics is not the cause, since the contraction rate of cancer of Chinese and Japanese women who moved to the West switched to the rate of the country they lived in within one or two generations.[38]

In his book Don't Drink Your Milk, Dr. Frank A. Oski, former director of the Department of Pediatrics at Johns Hopkins University School of Medicine and the Johns Hopkins Children Center, describes his findings on cow's milk and its effects in humans.

"I often wonder: Why are we the only mammal that drinks milk from another mammal that is not of its species? Why do we insist on never weaning?"

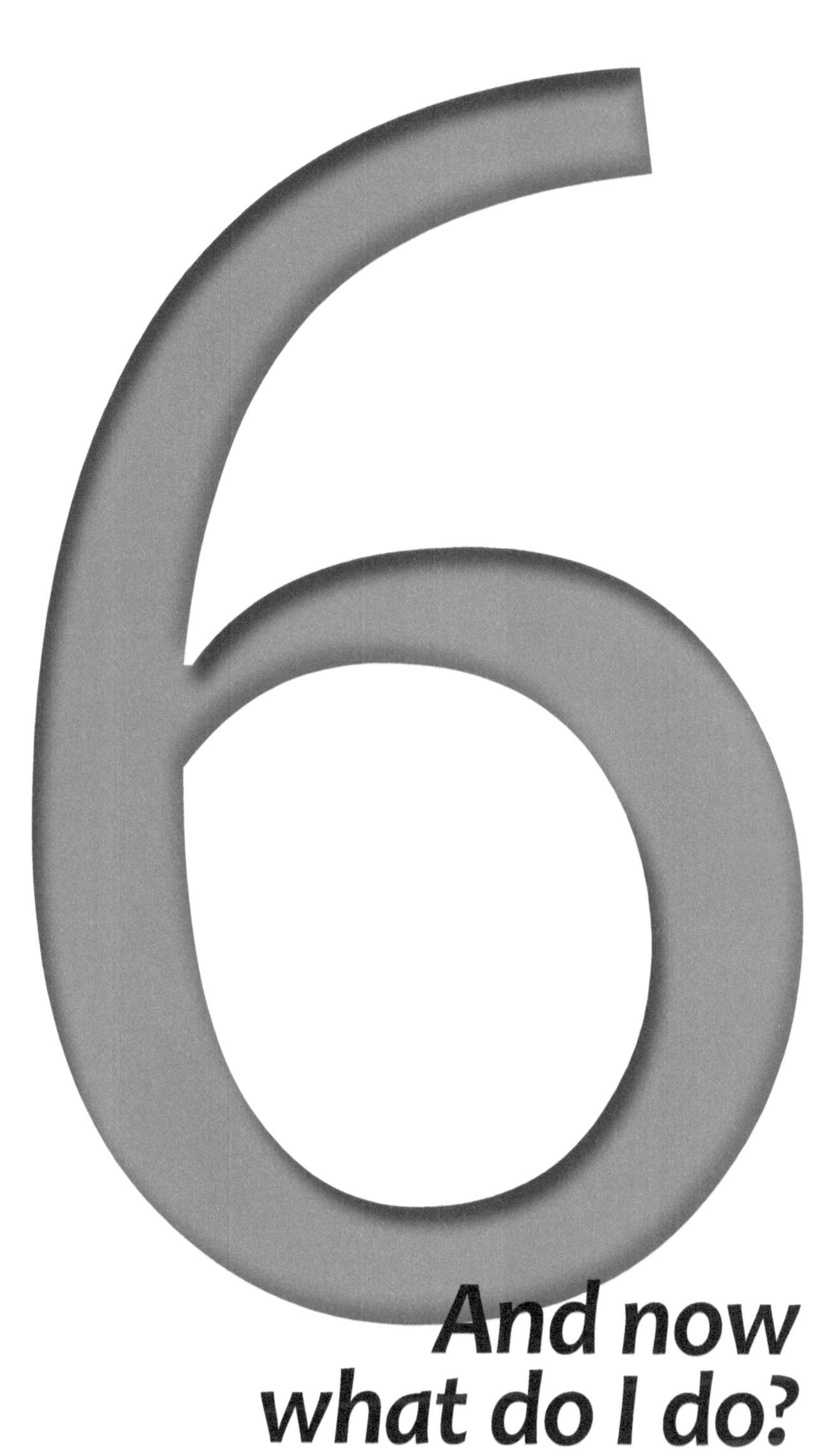

And now what do I do?

That's the question many mothers ask once they manage to identify the relationship of symptoms with the types of food that hurt their children. No one ever told us! Not even the doctors who only prescribe different medications to control symptoms without solving the core problem. Considering for the first time the possibility that what we eat may be the cause of repeated and continuous disease still seems incredible. Once you have found the types of foods that need to be eliminated from your diet, you will be surprised when, as if by magic, the symptoms disappear.

The temptation to go back to eating what we used to eat is a constant preoccupation. As we go through the test of reintroducing a specific food in the short term, we sometimes confirm that it is not the right time yet, and maybe we need a few more months. How do you know whether this is true? Your body will tell you.

I think in many ways we have failed to observe and listen. Whether its obesity or problems with anorexia, food is not only a factor that is essential to live, but it is a social and psychological issue by which we can comfort or punish ourselves. In all cultures and throughout history, family life revolves around a table. A birthday, a wedding, a baptism and even a funeral are reasons to sit down with family to eat. This means that food not only sustains us but it is also a reason to live and share. And what happens when someone breaks that pattern or alters in any way the family tradition? Worse, what happens when someone dares to blame any of the familiar menu items as the cause of their persistent discomfort? It is likely to unleash attacks and criticism from the family against the insurgent who dares to make such an accusation.

In my case, the faces of disbelief came quickly, along with an avalanche of well-intentioned opinions and comments, which did not help or make me feel understood. I realized that I should strive to follow the instructions that the new doctor had given me and follow what my intuition told me. I closed my ears to those who had no idea what we were living through at home and had no experience in the field. I began to observe and try new things. Albert Einstein once said that "if you always do the same thing, do not expect different results"; so I decided I had to try new things and expect different results as well.

That is what I tell mothers who write me and ask "now what do I do?" They already know the types of food that hurt their children, and they have understood that it is not only the job of the doctors and medicines, but also of themselves. The attitude we have in the face of this challenge is vital for success.

Here are some ideas that have worked for me and I'd like to share them with you:

1. *Take control:*

Every day there are more options to make food preparation easier; since our days are so busy, there is often no time to cook. At other times, we simply have no interest to do so, or do not know how. Take out grandma's recipe book, which has been forgotten in a drawer, and those delicious family recipes that have not surfaced in the last 20 years now the new generations can enjoy. It's time to take advantage of these simple recipes, which are not only nutritious but the ingredients are right there already. This is the opportunity to teach our children to try new and different flavors and introduce them to new foods. There is a world of flavors beyond chicken nuggets, quesadillas, and cereal with milk. And it's not just for the taste itself, but also for the nutrients that a varied diet can offer, taking advantage of the vitamins and minerals that food gives us.

Try to avoid prepared foods, as it will be difficult for you to identify all the ingredients they contain. When you go out to eat at restaurants, let the waiters know what foods you cannot eat so they can indicate what dishes do not contain the elements that harm you. Preferably choose dishes that are grilled or that are fresh. Avoid soups, salad dressings, and dishes with many ingredients.

The current diet of many children is full of sugars and dyes and lacking in vitamins, minerals, and proteins, which prevents us in being a healthy population this century. We have learned and gained a lot of ground in combating diseases of various kinds. We attack bacteria and viruses successfully, but it seems that when it comes to our diet we have taken a step back since we have exchanged fresh and recently prepared food for food that is frozen, fried, and sugary.

Women who are breastfeeding should know that the protein from cow's milk that they consume is passed through breast milk causing colic, reflux, and rhinitis in infants.[39] By eliminating dairy from your diet, you will notice an immediate change in your baby's symptoms.

2. *Read labels:*

If you read carefully the nutritional information on foods you buy, you will be surprised to discover that some of them contain ingredients that you did not expect. For example, fried corn tortillas may contain wheat and milk. Cereals contain ingredients that are difficult to decipher and many of them are preservatives, dyes, and sugars. The question is: What can be done to avoid these unsuspected ingredients?

Prepare your food yourself, especially at first when you are in the process of elimination and observation. The only way you can tell if a food is harmful to your children is if you know the foods they are eating and the reaction they have after eating them.

Cereals, crackers, juices, cold cuts, frozen food and sweets are some foods that I suggest avoiding, as they contain too many chemicals and an endless list of ingredients that are very difficult to translate and are often even difficult to pronounce.

I remember when I started the diet, which included eliminating wheat, I offered the children a box of cereal that was advertised as flakes of corn to be eaten without milk. I was convinced that they could eat it without any problems. I could not have been more wrong; the children had the same response, as always, with a runny nose and cough, so it was clear that the cereal also caused these reactions.

Coughing and a runny nose became clear signs of which foods my children tolerated and which foods they did not. In other cases, diarrhea, constipation, or intestinal inflammation will tell your body that some foods are not adequate.

Organic products have few ingredients and use no preservatives or artificial colors. Try to buy those products that have no more than 4 or 5 ingredients and make sure you know what each ingredient is. It is a simple way to eliminate products that can cause problems.

As consumers, we have the power to choose and eliminate what we dislike. Many companies have already realized that, and now there are more nutritious and healthy options to choose from. For example, you can choose between cereals in their more natural form such as oats, rice, lentils, chickpeas, quinoa and barley

3. Ignore criticism:

It is likely that on the road to recovery you will know people close to you who do not understand. With good intentions, they will kindly offer a list of recommendations that will only confuse you. They will often criticize you for the changes you're doing, your new way of eating, or be bothered because now you refuse food. They just do not understand. It's still happening to me all the time; after more than 6 years! There are still people who question our eating habits and start an endless debate about why we should eat dairy. What I do not understand is: Why should they care? Why are they so upset? Why do I have to explain myself to them?

For a long time I would go into detail about why we had to bring our own food or why we could not eat pizza; that bothered and exhausted me. I was tired of having to justify myself. My husband insisted that we did not have to talk about it and we could sit down and serve ourselves what we needed, without further comment. That's what we do now, and we are able to avoid many arguments and unhappy meals. It might be easier if I just answer, "I don't like it", but I usually reply that we cannot eat something, which is enough to unleash a barrage of questions.

I've learned that we should all be respectful of others, and to respect others style of eating, if they follow a special diet or eat just for the pleasure of it. We all believe we're always right, and what works for some does not work for others. Respect for the rights of others is peace, so it is said. So please ignore unwelcome comments and follow your instinct.

4. Be consistent:

Once you've decided to try a new style of eating and you see positive changes, it's just a matter of being persistent. It takes just one bite of a food that hurts you to trigger symptoms. You will need a few days to get over it or even a drug to diminish its effect. From what I've learned, it's not worth all the trouble to continue eating something that can hurt me. With your inner wisdom, you will try to avoid it as much as possible and thus save yourself all of these problems.

Children are wonderful and are also very wise; they do not want to feel bad. All you will need to do is remind them how bad they felt the last time they ate that food, and they will choose not to eat it on their own. You can offer them a substitute that they can eat to satisfy the craving.

Candies were eliminated from my children's diet. I tried to identify which candies sweets didn't harm them, but it was exhausting because I could not identify them exactly, so they got sick each time they ate them. Their pediatrician and I spoke with them before removing the candies from their diet, and they understood it perfectly. On Halloween we make a deal with our children; we agree to buy the biggest, most delicious sorbet or dessert they can eat. They can also dress up and ask for Halloween candy, only if when they return home that candy is re-used, so my kids enjoy giving their candy to their friends.

I'm sure you will also find new ways to celebrate and enjoy children's parties without anyone ending up in the hospital.

5. Expand your options:

Now is the opportunity to try new flavors and ingredients and even learn to cook. The possibilities are endless. There are a variety of foods such as grains, proteins from various sources that have not been tried before, fish, chickpeas, lentils, pomegranate, prickly pear, cactus, rabbit, cod, salmon, pumpkin, squash, beans, sardines, sweet potatoes, olives, almonds, fresh fruit juice, oatmeal, blueberries and so many other options.

I have seen many children limit their food choices and live with a very limited diet: some chicken, pasta, pizza, cereal, milk and, hopefully, a banana or an apple. Moms obey and respect their will, thus sparing them from coming across new flavors. By offering fun ways to do this and with more determination on our part, our children will have the opportunity to explore flavors, textures and, above all, different nutrients.

It is important that as mothers, responsible for our children's diet and health, we motivate them and find a way for them to have a more varied and enriched diet. Give them a taste of our "adult" dishes and be surprised to discover that they enjoy eating asparagus, pomegranate or mushrooms.

You can read in books or online for information about healthy food for children, discovering new ways to eat, and your family will be surprised with the new dishes. Salads and soups are an easy way to include several vegetables, and when placed with chicken or fish, they make a full meal. You could explore foods from other cultures, such as Japanese, Arabian, Indian and Chinese and thus expand your options.

6. *Water and Supplements:*

Both adults and children have forgotten to drink water. We are filled with soda or juices filled with dyes and sugars. I've seen babies drink soda in the bottle and teenagers drink milk like water. I've heard adults who confess that they only drink coffee and soda, not a glass of water. Our bodies are made mostly of water. We could live without food for several days, but no more than two days without water. Rediscover going back to the basics, which is indispensable to live, i.e. water. Get your children used to hydrating themselves with water instead of sports drinks or juices. What about you, have you discovered water?

The issue of dietary supplements is a complex one. It is best to talk to your doctor about whether you should include vitamin supplements in your diet as a vitamin deficiency can weaken your immune system. It is essential that you include vitamins in your daily meals.

7. See the glass as half full:

When you decide to stop eating something you like but that harms you, at first it can be very difficult. When I started reviewing the foods we could eat and comparing them with those we could not eat, I realized I was very wrong in my perception of feeling limited; we could eat much more than we imagined. It was only a matter of changing the approach. The problem is that I was used to including dairy in my meals, so in the beginning I thought it took away everything, when in reality, it allowed us to expand our diet, vary it, and enrich it.

Before, breakfast was cereal with milk; lunch, pasta with cream and chicken; and dinner, quesadillas. Now breakfast can consist of diced chicken and avocado; lunch, rice salad and grilled chicken; and dinner, tuna salad with vegetables. Not bad, right? Not eating less, but different.

So, why see the glass as half empty? List all the other foods you can eat and you will realize that it is not restrictive, but simply a different way of eating than the one you have right now. With this list, start looking for recipes that you enjoy, or adapt them, substituting one ingredient for another.

When you eat away from home

What I propose is more than a new diet but a different lifestyle. You may find it difficult to start, but soon you will discover that it is simple and easy. What sometimes remain are the questions and jokes about it, which you'll learn to ignore.

In developed countries like the U.S., the school systems have implemented a program for children with food allergies as there are very severe cases, particularly to peanuts, which can kill those who suffer from it. So depending on the degree of the allergy, it is possible to prevent not only the child who suffers from it, but also their classmates from eating food with this ingredient in order to minimize possible contact.

What I like is the dissemination and education on this subject, being informed and, above all, respect for people who suffer. Nobody looks at them weird or offers them food they cannot eat. This is also seen in sports teams, camps, and other activities involving children and food.

On a recent family vacation, we had a pleasant experience, which really impressed me, and I would like to share with you. It was on a trip to an amusement park in Florida. When making the reservations at restaurants inside the park, in addition to taking all our personal data, they asked if we had any restriction in our diet. I selected yes, dairy-free diet. I honestly did not know how much help would come from selecting it, but I decided to try.

The first restaurant we visited was a buffet. When we arrived at the table there was a ticket there with a note about the diet restriction. There was a very friendly waiter who explained that the chef would come to our table. The chef patiently accompanied us to the buffet and told us which dishes were dairy-free. Half of the buffet contained dishes we could eat. We were able to taste delicious dishes such as baked salmon, rice, roast beef, salads, rice, and baked potatoes. And they even went beyond our wildest expectations. The chef sent a special dessert to our table that was made especially for us: sorbet with soymilk and cookies without milk or gluten. We had to ask for more, and he kindly provided us a double portion. This attention was repeated at all of the buffet restaurants. In restaurants with food à la carte, the chef also visited us at the table and reviewed with us which dishes we could eat or, if necessary, they prepared something special. On one occasion we were surprised with a dairy- and gluten-free brownie, which was the best I've eaten in years.

In addition to the delicious food we ate, I want to make a special note of the attitude and the willingness of all of the staff who greeted us, made us feel understood and respected, and made our trip very special.

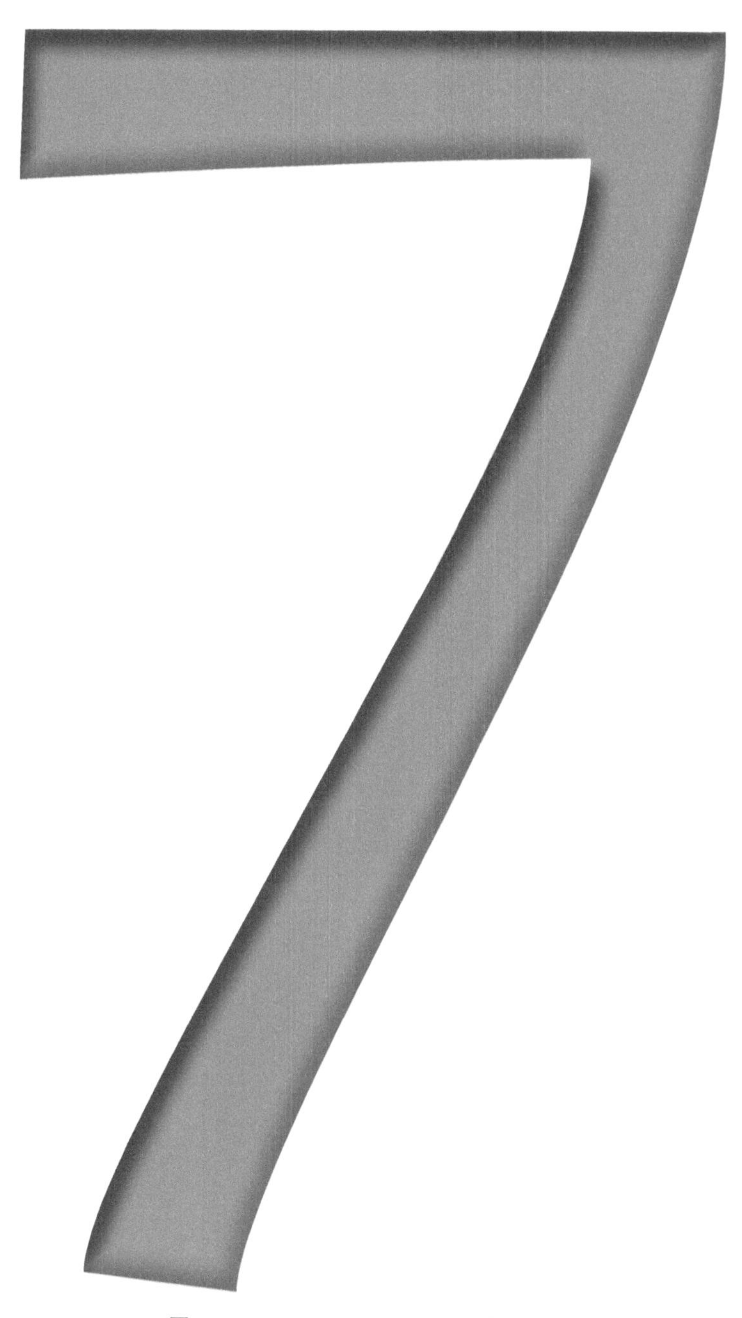

Among Moms

In this space I have included what other parents have learned as they have successfully overcome and managed this issue.

Luis´s Mothers:

I think it's important to assure yourself that your doctors are familiar with allergies so that they detect them early and know how to handle the situation in the best way. And if they are going to refer you to a specialist, make sure that there is good communication between them.

Be patient, as my other two children were also allergic, and now I know this is a process they will eventually overcome; do not despair! Be very strict with the diet, so that it may work. It is not easy, but it is not impossible either.

If there is one person I know who was patient with her children's allergies, it is Luis's mother. She has always worked hard and taken great care to give her children what they could eat at the time, with food prepared by her personally according to the needs of each child. She was sure that, with time and proper care, they would beat it. And that's exactly what happened.

Roberto´s Mother:

Listen to your intuition. I knew something was not

right with my son because my first daughter was always healthy, and I knew something was not right with Roberto, but no one could find the cause. Get several opinions and make the best decision listening to your intuition that as parents we develop, as we are the ones who know our children best.

Roberto's mother did not sit idly by or settle for what one doctor said. When I met her and we shared experiences, we mutually enriched each other and shared stories, tips, and doctors.

From her I learned that it is very important to keep medical records, keep track of the specialists who have been visited, tests that have been conducted with their results, and the medications administered.

Daniel and Lucía´s Mother:

If your baby starts to have unexplained diarrhea, remove the milk they are drinking, as they almost certainly are not tolerating the formula.

Daniel's experience had helped his mother lose no time in treating his sister, Lucia. Chances are that if a family member has allergies, another member may also have them.

Although there are many options for formula, none can equal breast milk as it is especially designed to feed human babies, contains all the nutrients the baby needs, is easily digested, and it's free. There is also La

Leche League, a group of nonprofit mothers who teach and provide support for nursing mothers.

Pablo´s Mother:

Do not waste time; act as quickly as possible. Following the diet to the letter is difficult, but not impossible. At any supermarket you can now find many specialty foods free of milk, gluten, nuts, etc.

Pablo's mother is very careful in feeding her children; she finds foods that contain no preservatives or colorings. She is always looking for tastier and more attractive options for her children. She confirmed the importance of being strict with adherence to the diet, as it contributed to improving Pablo's health.

Jorge´s Mother:

You must be convinced of the diagnosis and of following the right diet. It is very important that the family stand together and avoid eating foods that are outside of the diet. You must follow the diet strictly in order to see improvement. You are not the only ones with this problem; get informed about the issue and don't feel bad about taking away some food items from your children. It's for their own good, and they will understand later.

Jorge's mother is a doctor, and she realized that

the solidarity of the whole family was of great help to Jorge. Without this support, the road to recovery is very difficult.

Paola´s Mother:

If a child gets sick often and for a long time, I recommend you go to an allergist.

Believing that it is normal that our children are sick all the time simply because of their young age and the fact that they attend school where they come into contact with many bugs, is for me, a false premise. The frequency and duration of the illnesses should be checked to see if there is a problem.

Diego and Andrea´s Mother:

As a food engineer, I was able to realize that it is difficult to get rid of milk and dairy products, but now I know that not everyone tolerates these things the same way. Now, I too avoid these foods as well as processed foods.

Although we all believe that we eat a balanced and healthy diet, not everyone digests or assimilates all foods in the same way, so we must listen to our body when, through various mechanisms, it alerts us that something is not right. Let's listen to it.

Jennifer and Sam´s Mother:

"Do a food allergy panel and test for nutrients as well. Our final determination has been that our stainless steel copper core pots were leaching copper. Both kids' elevated copper levels could be contributing to their symptoms. We now have titanium water based cook wear, and give them an awful lot of zinc to counterbalance the copper until it naturally depletes itself. My son drips in sweat without the zinc and is up for hours through the night. I never run out of zinc.

I have also created allergy cards which go to all play dates. Friends, well intentioned parents who do not realize that corn is in many forms than just a kernel (such as corn starch, corn syrup and high fructose corn syrup), really cannot comprehend the 4-day temper tantrum that evolves as a result of my daughter eating something such as a brownie. I suggest fresh fruit and calling my cell phone should they wish to give them anything else. My dear friends love the cards and request one if they are taking the kids anywhere to eat. They hand it to the restaurant manager."

I am impressed with all the things and experience of this mother. I empathize immediately with her because when you realize for the first time that some foods can get you sick, and how your children's life and yours could change by just making an effort to change your diet, you will always be aware of what you eat and will always be aware of the related symptoms.

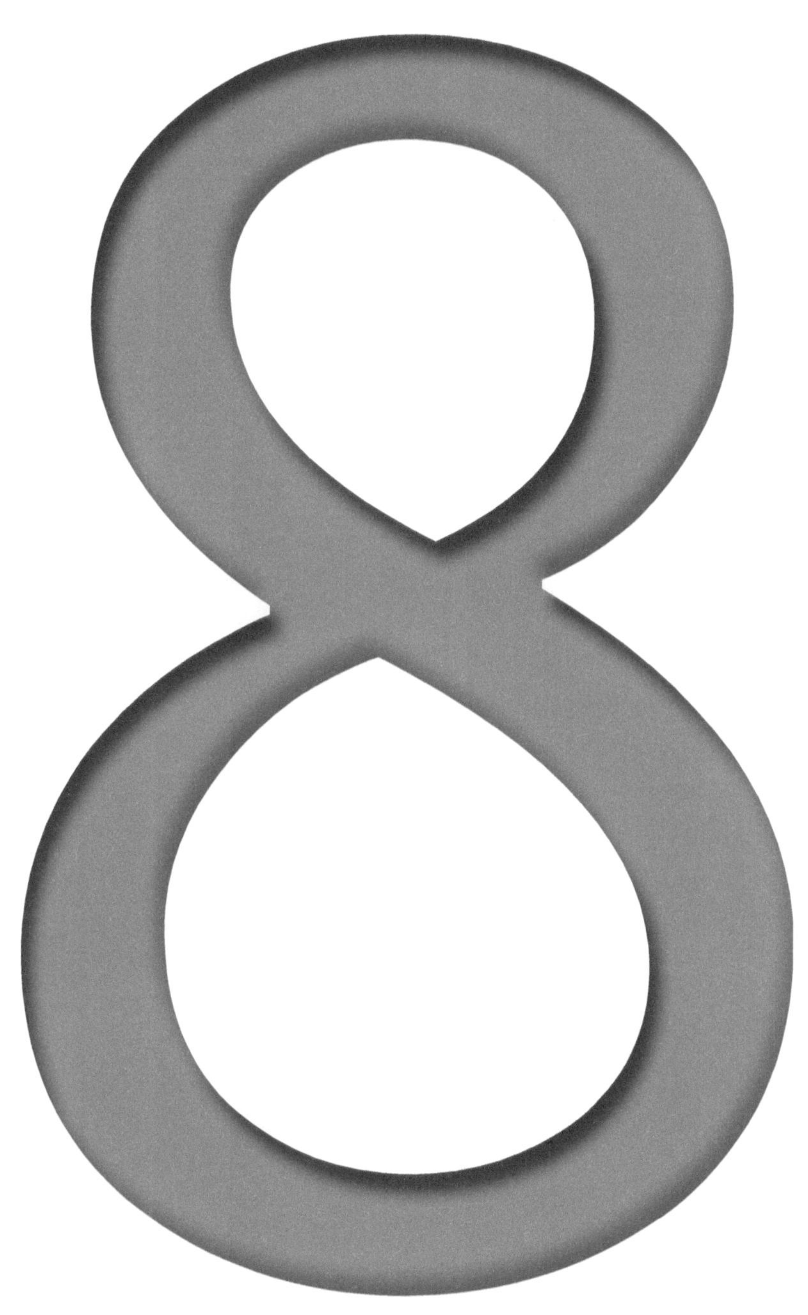

You are not alone

I have often wondered why it took so long to understand what was wrong with my children. Why did I have to consult so many doctors before learning that food allergies were able to disrupt the body so much that, over the years, they generate chronic diseases that are more difficult to treat and cure? I want to think it's because of ignorance and the complexity of the diagnosis. Since there are so many symptoms, a lot depends on the observation of the parents as well as the discipline and determination to follow a special diet.

To those who suffer from allergies, who take antihistamines throughout the year, who have children with asthma, or constantly have a runny nose, I recommend a milk-free diet. When I make this suggestion, I'm looked at with disbelief and am immediately told: "I could never give up milk". And when it comes to children, I'm told it can't be done because their diet is based on milk and wheat, and "children have to drink milk." My response to that is: there is a great variety of more nutritious foods that provide all the nutrients our bodies need. There are other foods that provide protein and calcium. When it comes to milk and in the case of other foods that should be excluded from the diet, there are other types of food able to provide the necessary nutrients. Therefore, it is important that a specialist monitors the diet to ensure it is properly balanced.

If this topic is so well documented in the medical journals, why are so many people undiagnosed? Or worse, why are so many people misdiagnosed?

Doctors also have a challenge: to see their patients as a whole being again, and not as a diseased organ or an isolated symptom. We ourselves have to take responsibility for our health, to follow the treatment properly, and seek second and third diagnoses if we are not satisfied with the one we receive. As parents, we know our children, and our parental intuition should lead us to know that we are doing the right thing.

Why are we not able to strictly follow a treatment or a diet? Why are we embarrassed to ask? Why do we settle for an answer that leaves us uneasy or dissatisfied?

For a long time I felt alone and misunderstood while caring for my sick children. Stress, anxiety, and guilt began to affect my temper. I was angry, frustrated, and moody all the time. Today I want to say you're not alone. In the previous chapter you read stories from other mothers who have been through the same situation. Now I will share stories from other people who shared their experiences with me after the first edition of this book was published in 2010.

Arturo is my friend Veronica's son. He began to have occasional stomach problems, complaining mainly of pain, without fever or temperature. The pain was more intense on some days than others, so she was puzzled and the doctor was unable to reach a diagnosis. He was visiting several doctors, including a pediatric gastroenterologist and an allergist, but they could not provide any answers. The pains continued to come and go, getting more and more intense, and they decided to perform an endoscopy, which was normal.

Veronica read the book, as she herself confesses, out of obligation. I hadn't seen her for a few months, and when we met again she told me now she knew what had been happening to Arturo. I was delighted for her and asked what the diagnosis was. "He is allergic to wheat." And how did she know? This is what she told me in her own words:

"For almost 5 years I went from one thing to another trying to find an answer to why my twins were always sick, either with a cold or a sore throat. And it was not until I talked with you that I realized how right you were when you told me not to dismiss the possibility that they might be allergic to certain foods. Thanks to your comment, I got them started on food and environment allergy tests.

The results of these tests did not yield particularly negative data with respect to the food. However, one of my children had already been complaining of stomach pain for about 9 months which at first was treated as gastritis, which was then discarded after an endoscopy, three biopsies (esophagus, stomach, and small intestine), and a gastric gammagram.

It was then when I decided to listen to you and to control the diet for both of my children. Even when the results of the tests weren't positive for dairy or wheat (only a little to melon, tobacco, and ash tree), the doctor's commented to me that oftentimes the chemical process by which certain foods are made are what causes discomfort for certain people. You recommended beginning a 'trial and error' diet with certain foods.

I spent many weeks 'removing and adding' foods which I believed were likely to harm them. I started with the most 'typical', moving to the least likely. And after a long struggle, I knew that my children's problem was bread (although allergy testing had been negative).

After this I went to an allergist who confirmed what you had often told me. In fact, my children could not tolerate the chemical process for wheat, so I removed it from their diet from that point forward.

Fortunately those ailments are over now, and after many years of giving antibiotics, which I often did not think were necessary, I found an answer to so many days of questions that often turned into frustration. Thank you very much.

Stories like my friend Veronica's began to happen to many people, so many and so unexpected that it never ceases to surprise me. This confirms the idea that everyone is different and that the effects of foods that harm us may be different too. Sometimes I'm asked, "But how is it that it didn't hurt you before and now it does?" And my answer is that there were so many symptoms of such a large variety (respiratory, stomach, vaginal) that they doctors never related them to the same source and much less with a type of food.

Francisco's case continues to surprise me; it makes me happy and confuses me at the same time. He is very close to me and very dear; a doctor by profession and vocation. All his life he suffered from allergies, and as a child he received vaccine treatments for many years.

As an adult, the runny nose and congestion persisted, this often got to be so severe that it caused vomiting. He also suffered from strong gastric reflux, which he had tried to confirm through tests, but the results were always negative. Everything seemed to indicate that he did not have reflux, but he had all the symptoms. That confused him even more. He eliminated things like hot and spicy foods from his diet without any improvement. He took various medications to get some relief but without much success. All these symptoms caused him to snore very loudly at night, and he could not do anything about it.

When he received a copy of this book, he took it very seriously without saying more. I think he thought how strange it was that I was talking about a health issue (since he's the doctor), but he read it nonetheless. A month later we met and he told me he had something important to tell me. I would never have imagined what I was going to hear next. He confided that he had eliminated dairy and wheat from his diet and felt like new; his symptoms had disappeared. He said he was not snoring; not at all, which I later confirmed with his wife. The reflux, as well as the rhinitis, had disappeared, after 50 years. After several days of having eliminated those foods, he confirmed that it was only the wheat that was the problem. I could not believe it, and I got really excited, especially to learn what he had discovered, to prove for himself that a food was causing him so much discomfort for so many years. As a physician, he could help more people in the same situation. And he has done so since.

A few months ago he shared with me that, while talking with colleagues, including gastroenterologists, he asked them how it was possible that they did not know more about food allergy and intolerance, and all the disorders that they can cause. Nobody said anything;

they could not answer. This only confirms the lack of information on all levels, both in society in general and on the part of health specialists.

I remember one of the e-mails I received in April 2010 after a local newspaper published a story about parents who researched and got involved in their children's illnesses. They wrote how the book had helped them, and how they had shared it with other families. This mom wrote:

I read the article from yesterday's Sunday paper, and I nearly fell out of my chair!

I read it early today, Monday, at 12:30 a.m., because I could not sleep because I have a 4 year old son who cannot stop coughing. He coughs all day, and just at that moment I grabbed the newspaper, because I could not sleep listening to him cough and cough; and I read the article. Right now it is 4:20 a.m., I went to your page to check the information on your book, which, of course, first thing tomorrow I am going to buy!

My son was diagnosed with reflux at 40 days old and had surgery. At a year and a half, he had bronchiolitis twice and thereafter it has been one consultation after another with doctors. I finally found an allergist who is treating him, but I still have not seen the results that I would like to see. My son is allergic to potatoes and tomatoes, plus dust, mites, and certain types of trees. I urgently need to know more, because my son's health is something that is affecting me emotionally. I cannot even sleep anymore because of his coughing, and I don't know what to do!

I cried when I read her letter because I was in a similar situation, and I understood the frustration and helplessness of not seeing your child improve despite all your efforts and those of physicians. With days that go by between doctor's visits, drugs, crying, runny nose, fever, vomiting, lab tests, insomnia, to start another cycle a few days later, with weak bodies, bags under the eyes, exhausted parents, poor school attendance, days of being locked indoors, midnight phone calls to the doctor, emergency room visits, just asking yourself: "When will it end?"

I know we are not the only ones. There are still many more families who cannot find an end to these constant symptoms. Many grow up this way, get used to suffering, but I have found that the changes I propose can mean a dramatic improvement in the quality of life for all involved, especially the children who suffer, as it is their growth, performance at school and even their behavior that is affected and compromised. There is no doubt that a sick child who feels bad most of the time, is not sleeping, and is taking lots of medication, can be irritable, dispersed, sleepy, grumpy, and distracted; don't you think?

If the doctor you currently see has not yet been able to help, perhaps it is time to look elsewhere, to try new ideas, to find a doctor who knows more about allergies.

I tried; I had nothing to lose. I did not ask the pediatrician that we saw at the time because he had expressed his view that my children's problem was not allergies. He saw only the immediate symptom and I needed a comprehensive solution to find the source of the problem.

Open yourself up to a new idea; give yourself and your children the opportunity to try something different, different medicines, antibiotics, nasal sprays and nebulizers. Read, document, and ask. I know you're not a doctor, but you're the mother of your children, and no one knows them better. You're the only one who can say that something is wrong, that the frequency of their illnesses is not normal. Do not give up, you must persevere.

Although there is a great deal of literature and many studies, the experiences of many families, when it comes to allergies, are difficult, long, and complex. It is clear that, ultimately, we are responsible for our health. What do you eat? What are you filling yourself with? Is it ignorance or apathy? It's your body, it's your health, and it's your decision. You have the opportunity to free yourself from the medication and unnecessary tests; you have the opportunity to have a healthy life.

Learning to listen to what our bodies tell us through a variety of symptoms will help us better care for it and allow us to give it what it needs. Your wisdom and intuition are there to help you. A healthy life is worth every effort, and to see your children healthy is priceless. Any road that is necessary to travel to improve their health is our responsibility, and is worth the effort. The smile on their faces will say it all.

ANNEXES

Annexe A

Accession Number:	**A0601250096**
Reference Number:	
Patient:	Alejandra Gutierrez
Age: 4	*Sex:* F
Date of Birth:	11/30/2001
Date Collected:	1/24/06
Date Received:	1/25/06
Report Date:	1/27/06
Telephone:	9253773000
Fax:	9256317948
Reprinted:	
Comment:	

0075 IgGI & 4 Food Antibodies (90 Antigens) Testing Performed by Metametrix,Inc., 4855 Peachtree Ind Blvd, Norcross, GA 30092 *Methodology: ELISA*

	Results		Class
Dairy/Meat/Poultry			
Beef	< 25		
Casein	< 25		
Chicken	< 25		
Egg, White	1,195	Severe	+5
Egg, Yolk	1,036	Severe	+5
Lamb	< 25		
Milk	56		
Pork	< 25		
Turkey	< 25		
Fish/Shellfish			
Clam	< 25		
Codfish	< 25		
Crab	< 25		
Flounder	< 25		
Halibut	< 25		
Lobster	< 25		
Mackerel	< 25		
Oyster	< 25		
Trout	< 25		
Salmon	< 25		
Shrimp	< 25		
Tuna	< 25		
Fruits			
Apple	< 25		
Banana	461	Moderate	+3
Blueberry	< 25		
Cantaloupe	< 25		
Cranberry	< 25		
Apricot	< 25		
Grape	< 25		
Grapefruit	< 25		
Honeydew	< 25		
Lemon	< 25		
Orange	< 25		
Peach	< 25		
Pear	< 25		
Pineapple	< 25		
Strawberry	< 25		
Watermelon	< 25		
Grains			
Barley	< 25		
Corn	< 25		
Oat	< 25		
Rice	< 25		
Rye	< 25		
Wheat	< 25		
Legumes			
Pea, Green	< 25		
Lentil	< 25		
Lima Bean	< 25		
Navy Bean	< 25		
Peanut	< 25		

	Results	Class
Pinto Bean	< 25	
Soybean	< 25	
Bean, String	< 25	
Miscellaneous		
Aspergillus	< 25	
Black Pepper	< 25	
Chocolate	51	
Cinnamon	< 25	
Coffee	< 25	
Ginger	< 25	
Malt	< 25	
Tea	< 25	
Vanilla	35	
Yeast, Baker's	30	
Yeast, Brewer's	33	
Nuts/Seeds		
Almond	36	
Cashew	< 25	
Coconut	< 25	
Pecan	< 25	
Pistachio	< 25	
Sesame	55	
Sunflower	54	
Walnut	< 25	
Vegetables		
Avocado	< 25	
Broccoli	< 25	
Cabbage	< 25	
Carrot	< 25	
Celery	< 25	
Cauliflower	< 25	
Cucumber	< 25	
Asparagus	< 25	
Garlic	< 25	
Lettuce	< 25	
Mushroom	< 25	
Mustard Greens	47	
Olive	< 25	
Onion	< 25	
Pepper, Green	< 25	
Spinach	< 25	
Sweet Potato	< 25	
Potato	< 25	
Tomato	< 25	
Zucchini	< 25	

Class Definitions:	Class	Cutoffs+
	Negative	0-75
	Mild (+1)	76-150
	Moderate (+2/+3/+4)	300/500/800
	Severe (+5)	801or more

These test results are not for the diagnosis of disease. They are intended to provide nutritional guidelines to qualified healthcare professionals with full knowledge of patient history and concerns to assist in their design of an appropriate healthcare program.

Georgia Lab Lic. Code #067-007
CLIA ID# 11D0255349

New York Clinical Lab PFI #4578
Florida Clinical Lab Lic. #800008124

Laboratory Directors J. Alexander Bralley, PhD
Robert M. David, PhD

Annexe B

PRUEBAS CUTANEAS

NOMBRE Gutierrez Gonzalez Alejandra M. EDAD 3 FECHA 4-Abril-05 P C D ✓ P. K.

TESTIGO DERMOGRAFISMO

POLENES

1.- AMBROSIA
2.- ARTEMISIA
3.- FRANSERIA
4.- XANTHIUM
5.- CAPRIOLA
6.- HOLCUS
7.- LOLIUM
8.- BROMUS
9.- AMARANTHUS
10.- ATRIPLEX
11.- CHENOPODIUM
12.- SALSOLA
13.- HELIANTHUS
14.- PLANTAGO
15.- SABINA
16.- FRAXINUS
17.- POPULUS ++
18.- MEZQUITE
19.- NOGAL
20.- ENCINO
21.- SAUCE
22.- TRUENO
23.- MAIZ

INHALANTES

1.- EP. GATO
2.- EP. PERRO
3.- EP. CONEJO
4.- EP. RES
5.- PLUMAS DE POLLO
6.- ALGODON
7.- LANA
8.- SEDA
9.- TABACO
10.- SEMILLA ALGODON
11.- POLVO DE CASA ++
12.- ACAROS

HONGOS

1.- ALTERNARIA
2.- HORMODENDRUM
3.- RHIZOPUS
4.- MUCOR
5.- TRINCHODERMA
6.- MONILIA A
7.- ASPERGILLUS

CONT.

8.- PENICILLIUM
9.- FUSARIUM
10.- PHOMA
11.- HELMINTOSPORIUM
12.- ESTREPTOMICES
13.- VAC. BACTERIANA

ALIMENTOS

1.- ARROZ
2.- CEBADA
3.- MAIZ
4.- TRIGO
5.- C. DE CERDO
6.- CHILE
7.- FRIJOL
8.- HUEVO CLARA
9.- HUEVO YEMA
10.- LECHE DE VACA
11.- QUESO
12.- SARDINA
13.- OSTION
14.- SOYA
15.- HISTAMINA ++++

CONT.

16.- CAMARON
17.- CAFE ++
18.- COCOA
19.- LEVADURA

FRUTAS

1.- AGUACATE
2.- CACAHUATE
3.- FRESA
4.- LIMON
5.- NARANJA
6.- PIÑA
7.- PLATANO
8.- MANGO

VERDURAS

1.- CEBOLLA
2.- LECHUGA
3.- PAPA
4.- PEPINO
5.- TOMATE
6.- ZANAHORIA
7.- OTROS

Annexe C

AGS (+)	No. FCO.	CONC.	FECHA
	5cc	Vacuna	Bacteriana.
	(1er Ciclo)	04. Abr. 05	
	(2do. Ciclo)	03. Jun. 05	
	(3er Ciclo)	29. JUL. 05	

TOS
DISNEA
SIBILANCIAS
EXPECTORACION

PRURITO
RINORREA
ESTORNUDOS
CONJUNTIVITIS

PAPULAS
ERITEMA
PRURITO
EDEMA
LABIO
PARPADO

BIBLIOGRAPHICAL REFERENCES

1. The food allergy and anaphylaxis network, www.foodallergy.org.

2. Gera en 56 Num 3 Mayo-Junio 2009.

3. Alergia E Inmunológica. Temas de Pediatría. Asociación Mexicana de Pediatría, A.C. 1997.

4. L. Kathleen Mahan, Sylvia Escott-Stump, Nutrición y Dietoterapia de Krause, Ninth Edition.

5. A. Malet Casajuana, Manual de Alergia Alimentaria para atención primaria, Masson, S.A. 1995.

6. Konrad Kail and Bobbi Lawrence, Allergy Free. An Alternative Medicine Definitive Guide, AlternativeMedicine.com Books, 2000.

7. L. Kathleen Mahan, Sylvia Escott-Stump, Nutrición y Dietoterapia de Krause, Ninth Edition.

8. Konrad Kail and Bobbi Lawrence, Allergy Free. An Alternative Medicine Definitive Guide, AlternativeMedicine.com Books, 2000.

9. Ranjit Kumar Chandra, Food Intolerance, 1984

10. Alergia a alimentos. Guia para su diagnóstico y tratamiento. Colegio Mexicano de Alergia, Asma e Inmunologia Pediatrica (COMAAIPE) www.compedia.org.mx.

11. Ibid.

12. The food allergy and anaphylaxis network, www.foodallergy.org.

13. Dr. Julio I. Mendez de Inocencio, Alergia, enfermedad multisistemica, Editorial Medica Panamericana, 2008.

14. Konrad Kail and Bobbi Lawrence, Allergy Free. An Alternative Medicine Definitive Guide, Alternative-Medicine.com Books, 2000.

15. Ranjit Kumar Chandra, Food Intolerance, 1984.

16. Maurice E. Shils, Modern Nutrition in Health and Disease, Lippincott Williams & Wilkins, 2006.

17. Alergia a alimentos. Guia para su diagnóstico y tratamiento. Colegio Mexicano de Alergia, Asma e Inmunologia Pediatrica (COMAAIPE) www.compedia.org.mx.

18. Gerardo López Pérez, "Prevalencia de las enfermedades alergicas en la ciudad de México", Revista Alergia México volumen 56 Num 3 Mayo-Junio 2009

19. Ibid

20. Gerardo López Pérez, "Prevalencia de las enfermedades alergicas en la ciudad de México", Revista Alergia México volumen 56 Num 3 Mayo-Junio 2009.

21. Carlos M. Arroyave Hernandez, "Food Allergy Mediated by IgG Associated with Migraine in Adults", Revista Alergia México volume 54, Num. 5 Sept-Oct 2007.

22. Dr. Julio I. Mendez de Inocencio, Alergia, enfermedad multisistemica, Editorial Medica Panamericana, 2008.

23. Alergia a alimentos. Guia para su diagnóstico y tratamiento. Colegio Mexicano de Alergia, Asma e Inmunologia Pediatrica (COMAAIPE) www.compedia.org.mx.

24. Questionnaire for "Luis's" Mother's Testimony

25. Questionnaire for "Roberto's" Mother's Testimony

26. Questionnaire for "Daniel and Lucía's" Mother's Testimony

27. Questionnaire for "Pablo's" Mother's Testimony

28. Questionnaire for "Jorge's" Mother's Testimony

29. Questionnaire for "Paola's" Mother's Testimony

30. Questionnaire for "Diego and Andrea's" Mother's Testimony

31. Dr. Olga Cuevas Fernández, El equilibrio a través de la alimentación, Sorles SL León, 1999.

32. The food allergy and anaphylaxis network, www.foodallergy.org.

33. P.S. Papageorgiou, Clinical Aspects of Food Allergy, Biochemical Society, 2002.

34. Alergia a alimentos. Guia para su diagnóstico y tratamiento. Colegio Mexicano de Alergia, Asma e Inmunologia Pediatrica (COMAAIPE) www.compedia.org.mx.

35. Ross G. Crittenden Ph. D., Cow's Milk Allergy: A Complex Disorder, Journal of the American College of Nutrition, Vol. 24 No. 6, 582S-591S (202005).

36. Ibid

37. Dr. Olga Cuevas Fernández, El equilibrio a través de la alimentación, Sorles SL León, 1999.

38. Dr. Robert Cohen, Milk , the Deadly Poison, Argus Publishing, 1997

39. Jane A. Plant, Ph.D., Your Life in Your Hands, Thomas Dunne Books, 2001.

40. Ross G. Crittenden Ph. D., Cow's Milk Allergy: A Complex Disorder, Journal of the American College of Nutrition, Vol. 24 No. 6, 582S-591S (202005).

ACKNOWLEDGEMENTS

To my parents and my extended family for their unconditional love and all their wisdom.

To my in-laws, for their continued support and for making me part of their family.

To Monica and Imelda for their advice and contributions to this book.

Dr. Gerardo Velazquez for his valuable contribution.

To all the families who shared their valuable experience and confidence.

To all the doctors who dared to look beyond.

To Lula for helping me see the light.

To Vicky for her advice.

To Felipe and Victor for their contributions and literary recommendations.

To La Sociedad, for publicity and advertising of the cover and for its valuable advice.

To all who have supported me during this project, for your words and your faith.

To Carmen for your help and advices in this English version.

To Martanelly for your beautiful work in the interior design.

Sites of Interest:

NotMilk:
www.notmilk.com

The Food Allergy & Anaphylaxis Network:
www.foodallergy.org

American Academy of Allergy, Asthma & Immunology:
www.aaaai.org

SLaai:
www.slaai.org

Mexican Association of Pediatric Specialists in Allergy and Clinical Immunology:
www.compedia.org.mx

Alergia Alimentaria.org:
www.alergialimentaria.org

Jane Plant
www.janeplant.com

Celiac Disease & Gluten-free Diet Information

About the Author

Maria Alejandra Gonzalez graduated from the Tecnologico de Monterrey, with degrees in Marriage and Family Sciences and in Human Development.

She is a wife and the mother of 3 children.

www.ingramcontent.com/pod-product-compliance
Lightning Source LLC
Chambersburg PA
CBHW030346290526
45785CB00004B/1613
* 9 7 8 1 4 7 9 1 2 4 9 0 9 *